Biomedical Bestiary

An Epidemiologic Guide to Flaws and Fallacies in the Medical Literature

BIOMEDICAL BESTIARY

MAX MICHAEL III, M.D.
Chairman, Department of Medicine, The Cooper Green Hospital; Clinical Assistant Professor of Medicine, The University of Alabama School of Medicine, Birmingham, Alabama

W. THOMAS BOYCE, M.D.
Assistant Professor, Department of Pediatrics, University of Arizona College of Medicine, Tucson, Arizona

ALLEN J. WILCOX, M.D., Ph.D.
Medical Officer, Epidemiology Branch, National Institute of Environmental Health Sciences, Research Triangle Park, North Carolina

Drawings of beasts by Betsy Fleenor
Other line art by Marie Weaver

LITTLE, BROWN AND COMPANY
BOSTON/TORONTO

First Edition

Library of Congress Catalog Card No. 83-82941

ISBN 0-316-56951-8

Printed in the United States of America

FF

FOR MARILYN, FOR JILL, AND FOR CLAIRE

Contents

Preface

Most medical students regard epidemiology as somewhere between mud-wrestling and mah-jongg in its relevance to medicine. The worth of epidemiologic principles becomes more apparent later, when as physicians they begin to grapple with the imperfect evidence and conflicting conclusions of medical literature.

There are excellent textbooks available to medical students and clinicians who are interested in acquiring epidemiologic skills. Some of these are listed in the bibliography at the end of this book. Such twelve-course banquets are fine when you have the time, but there is also a place for fast food. What we offer here is a quick introduction to epidemiologic ideas in a format meant to be appetizing and easily digestible. We've sacrificed the more subtle seasonings, but not the nutritive value. If you should find yourself in the mood for more gourmet fare, references to fuller discussions of the epidemiologic issues involved are provided at the end of each chapter.

M. M.

W. T. B.

A. J. W.

Acknowledgments

This book has been influenced by many people. We wish to gratefully acknowledge the contributions of Russell Alexander, Kirk Avent, Ted Colton, Curt Eshelman, Walter Rogan, Jeff Roseman, Dale Sandler, Robert Sandler, Cathy Schaefer, and Ed Wagner.

Ideas for some of the chapters came from the original skit "Clinical Flaw Catching" created by the Clinical Scholars at the University of North Carolina. The impetus for this book comes in part from the work of Earl Bryant, Phil Compeau, and Russ Ward.

Our special thanks to Dave McKay for his ongoing support and for his substantive editorial comments.

We are also indebted to Pam Doss and Deb Zeman for their tireless secretarial support.

Finally, we would like to acknowledge our constant debt to our teacher, the late John Cassel, whose zest for this subject was abundant and contagious.

Introduction

Medical research is full of fiends and goblins who distort clinical measurements, disrupt protocols, and cloud the processes of logic. These demons cheerfully infest the medical literature. They leer unabashedly from behind "Materials and Methods" sections, gaily pollute "Results," and wreak havoc with "Conclusions." Goblin-catching marvels like the randomized clinical trial or logistic regression analysis are some defense. But, alas, each defense also provides new nooks and crannies for monsters to haunt.

We present a bestiary of these creatures, describing their quirks, their charms, and their haunts. Bestiaries originated in the second century as fanciful catalogs of the animal kingdom. Our bestiary explores the more modern territory of biomedical research. It describes the strange and wily beasts that lurk, sallow and yellow-eyed, in the most respectable medical studies. With some foreknowledge of the creatures you might encounter, you can be more alert on your forays into the medical literature, more careful in your scientific thinking, and more able in your assessment of the strengths of medical research.

Each chapter begins with a description of a beast and a definition of the problem to be discussed. This is followed by one or two case reports. Most of these reports are fictitious, but the problems are real, as shown in the subsequent comments and examples. Each chapter closes with further real-life examples and references to more complete discussions of the problem.

One note of warning: These beasts have two sorts of victims—those who fail to see them, and those who can *only* see them. A beast-free scientific paper is as improbable as a germ-free handshake. Beasts are a part of the natural ecology. The challenge is to know what they are, where they are, and how to contain the damage they do.

Lastly, animal stories are to be enjoyed. Welcome to our zoo!

"And now," cried Max, "Let the wild rumpus start!"

Maurice Sendak
Where the Wild Things Are

Biomedical Bestiary

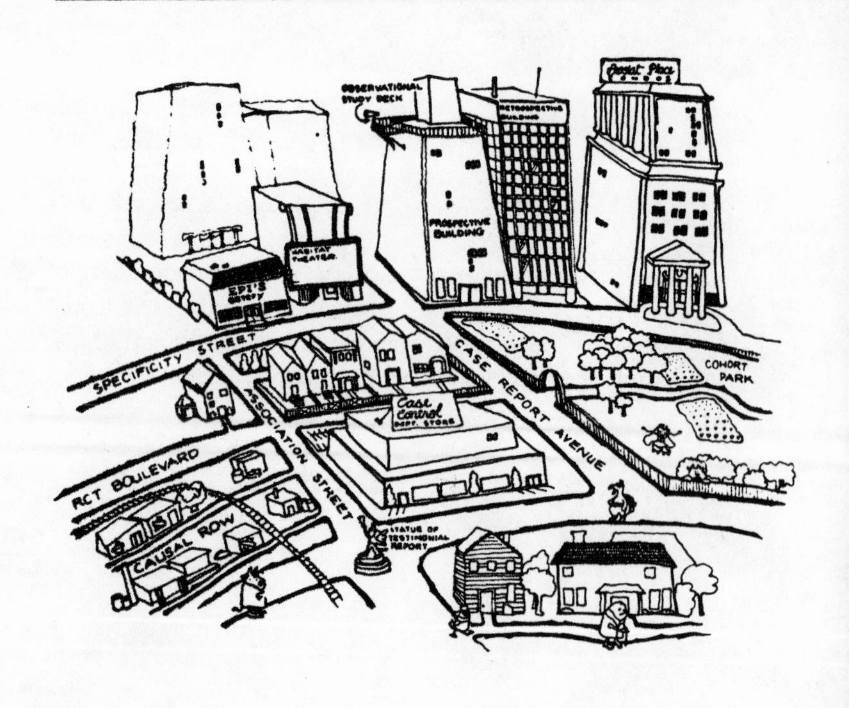

OBSERVATIONAL STUDY DECK
RETROSPECTIVE BUILDING
PROSPECTIVE BUILDING
HABITAT THEATER
EPI'S
SPECIFICITY STREET
CASE REPORT AVENUE
COHORT PARK
ASSOCIATION STREET
Case Control DEPT. STORE
RCT BOULEVARD
CAUSAL ROW
STATUE OF TESTIMONIAL REPORT

HABITATS
An Overview of Study Designs

The purpose of most medical research is to find causes of disease and ways to prevent or treat disease. To that end scientists have devised an ingenious assortment of strategies and research designs. Some are as simple as the astute observation of a new disease. Others are complex and expensive, such as the clinical trial. Each research design has made contributions to our understanding of disease. At the same time, no strategy provides foolproof answers. Each has its own peculiar strengths and limits, and each provides refuge to gremlins who will twist conclusions and lead us astray.

In this chapter, we briefly describe the major research study designs. These study designs are something like neighborhoods: their boundaries aren't distinct, but each has its own special flavor. Furthermore, each attracts certain sorts of residents. If you can identify the neighborhood you're in as you read the medical literature, you'll have a better idea of what kind of beast you're likely to run into.

EXPERIMENTAL STUDIES

Definition: An experimental study is distinguished by the fact that members of a study population are assigned to either a treatment or control group. The treated and untreated groups are then followed prospectively to see whether the two groups subsequently differ.

Experimental studies are the high-rent district of medical research. Experimental designs, such as the double-blind randomized controlled clinical trial, are the type of human research most analogous to experiments done in the laboratory. The resemblance of this study design to formal bench research gives it a certain prestige. Nonetheless, there are limitations even to this research strategy. First, it is expensive. There are not enough resources to permit every interesting question to be studied with such a design. Another limitation is that some important questions cannot be addressed by the experimental trial. Rare effects, such as the occurrence of Guillain-Barré syndrome following swine influenza vaccination, can require many thousands of persons to be exposed before the effect is detected. For cases in which the effect of interest is a harmful one, no experimental trial of any size can be ethically justified. These cases include such questions as the toxic effect of food additives, waste chemicals, or low-level radiation. Finally, even experimental designs are susceptible to bias and misinterpretation. The most airtight randomized trial cannot totally regulate the behavior of its participants or investigators. Many of the beasts have found comfortable niches in the neighborhood of experimental studies at one time or another.

OBSERVATIONAL STUDIES

Definition: An observational study is one in which the treatment or exposure of interest is not assigned, but instead occurs by choice or by happenstance.

Observational studies depend on people's natural or voluntary exposures to factors that ordinarily cannot be randomly assigned. Examples of such factors are cigarette smoking or employment in a uranium mine. In the experimental study design discussed previously, the factor under study is randomly assigned, so that members of the study and control groups are otherwise similar. In contrast, there is always the possibility in observational studies that the exposed and unexposed groups differ in important ways other than exposure—ways that may affect the risk of subsequent disease. This possibility must constantly be taken into account when conducting and interpreting observational studies.

Observational studies encompass most of the territory of epidemiologic research. The sheer variety of the terrain makes for an assortment of beastly nesting places. Here are the major neighborhoods.

The Case Report

Definition: A case report describes a small number of persons with an unusual disease or an unusual change in their disease that is possibly related to a single cause.

Case reports are usually the first statement of a clinical hypothesis. In this manner, the alert clinician provides the grist for much epidemiologic research. Many important discoveries have started with a clinician who spotted an unusual pattern of disease. The detection by physicians of an unusual cluster of vaginal cancers led to the discovery that diethylstilbestrol is a transplacental carcinogen. Physicians specializing in occupational medicine helped to identify vinyl chloride as a carcinogen when they recognized the above-average rates of occurrence of a rare liver tumor among chemical workers. However, while case reports may lead to important findings, they cannot usually be regarded as a finding in themselves because the observation may be due to chance.

The Cross-Sectional Study

Definition: A cross-sectional study (also known as a survey or prevalence study) looks for an association between a disease and its possible causes by studying the characteristics of a group of people at one point in time.

This design can demonstrate an association between a factor and a disease, but it doesn't necessarily show which came first. For example, a census of elderly people may show that there are more people with hip fractures living in nursing homes than in their own homes. Does this mean nursing homes are a more dangerous place to live? Or do people with hip fractures go to nursing homes? The cross-sectional study is appropriate for preliminary explorations but it cannot provide definite answers. The advantage of the cross-sectional study is that it is relatively inexpensive and easy to perform.

The Ecologic Study

Definition: The ecologic study (also known as an aggregate or descriptive study) uses data that are routinely collected for various purposes to study the occurrence of a disease and its possible causes among groups of groups.

Most epidemiologic studies collect data from individuals. However, it is possible to compare groups of groups (e.g., groups of countries, states, or counties) in order to investigate possible causes of disease. For example, heart disease may be shown to be more common in people living in countries where high-fat diets are the norm than in people living in countries where low-fat diets prevail. From this it might be inferred that individuals with high-fat diets are at greater risk for heart disease.

Ecologic studies can be cross-sectional, as in the example above, or they can look at changes over time. The advantage of ecologic studies is that they use data that are routinely collected and already available, making the study relatively inexpensive. Like the cross-sectional design, it is most appropriate for preliminary exploratory studies. Inferences drawn from the study of groups are not necessarily true for individuals (see Chapter 12, Ecologic Fallacy). Findings from this type of study require confirmation by other study designs.

The Case-Control Study

Definition: A case-control study (also known as a case-history or case-referent study) is one that begins with study subjects (cases) who have the disease of interest and a comparison group without the disease. Then the previous exposures of both groups are investigated. If a previous exposure is more common among the ill group, this is regarded as evidence that the exposure caused the disease.

The case-control approach differs from other observational designs in that the investigation begins with persons who are already sick and works back to document possible causes of their illness. In a sense this approach is a refinement of the case report, in which the alert practitioner observes one or more persons with a particular illness. In the case-control study, this observation is refined by adding a group of persons who do not have the illness, and then comparing the two groups in terms of their previous exposures. The case-control design is relatively efficient, especially for rare diseases. However, it raises methodologic questions that confuse even the experts. For example, it is not clear by what criteria the comparison group should be chosen (see Chapter 14, Matchmaker).

The Cohort Study

Definition: A cohort study (also known as a follow-up, incidence, or panel study) is one in which the researcher starts with one group of persons exposed to a factor of interest and another comparable group that is unexposed. These groups are then observed at a later time to see if they have developed differences that might be attributable to their different exposures.

Cohort studies are often prospective; that is, subjects are identified and then followed over time. However, a cohort study can also be retrospective, in the sense that it uses data collected in the past. For example, a researcher may use occupational records to identify groups of people who were exposed to a substance thirty years previously, and then trace those persons to the present to observe subsequent health effects.

The prospective cohort study is the type of observational study most resembling the experimental design. In both the cohort and the experimental study the experience of exposed and unexposed persons is studied over time. This permits careful measurement of an effect where one exists, although usually at considerable expense.

DIAGNOSTIC TESTS

In addition to studying the cause and treatment of disease, physicians must develop and evaluate the tools they use to identify disease. The evaluation of diagnostic tests is a small research neighborhood, but includes some unique problems of logical inference; as will be seen.

We have described several neighborhoods of research designs. Now you will be introduced to the beasts who call these neighborhoods home. Some of the beasts are very fussy about where they hang out. Berkson Bias, for example, wouldn't be caught dead outside the case control district. Others roam freely with utter disregard for neighborhood boundaries. This guide suggests in which study neighborhoods the beasts are most likely to be found.

We have described several neighborhoods of research designs. Now you will be introduced to the beasts who call these neighborhoods home. Some of the beasts are very fussy about where they hang out. Berkson Bias, for example, wouldn't be caught dead outside the case control district. Others roam freely with utter disregard for neighborhood boundaries. This guide suggests in which study neighborhoods the beasts are most likely to be found.

A GUIDE TO THE BEASTS AND THEIR HAUNTS

In most research neighborhoods

Grand Confounder: The possibility of alternative explanations (also known as confounding)
Numerator Monster: Issue of the missing denominator
Selection Bias: Bias in incomplete data
Response Bias: Bias in inexact data
Variable Observer: Even experts can disagree
Hawthorne Effect: The observer changes the observed
Diagnostic Accuracy Bias: Bias in the art of diagnosis
Regression Meany: Extremes approach the average (also known as regression to the mean)
Significance Turkey: Significant, but not important
Nerd of Nonsignificance: Important, but not significant

In cross-sectional studies

Cohort Effect: Interpreting an age effect

In ecologic studies

Ecologic Fallacy: Inferences from grouped data

In case-control studies

Berkson Bias: Selection bias in hospital-based studies
Matchmaker: Finding the right comparison group (also known as over- or under-matching)

In studies of diagnostic tests

Test Bloater: Disease prevalence and test usefulness
Diagnostic Zealot: Problems in judging new tests (also known as work-up and spectrum bias)

THE BEASTS

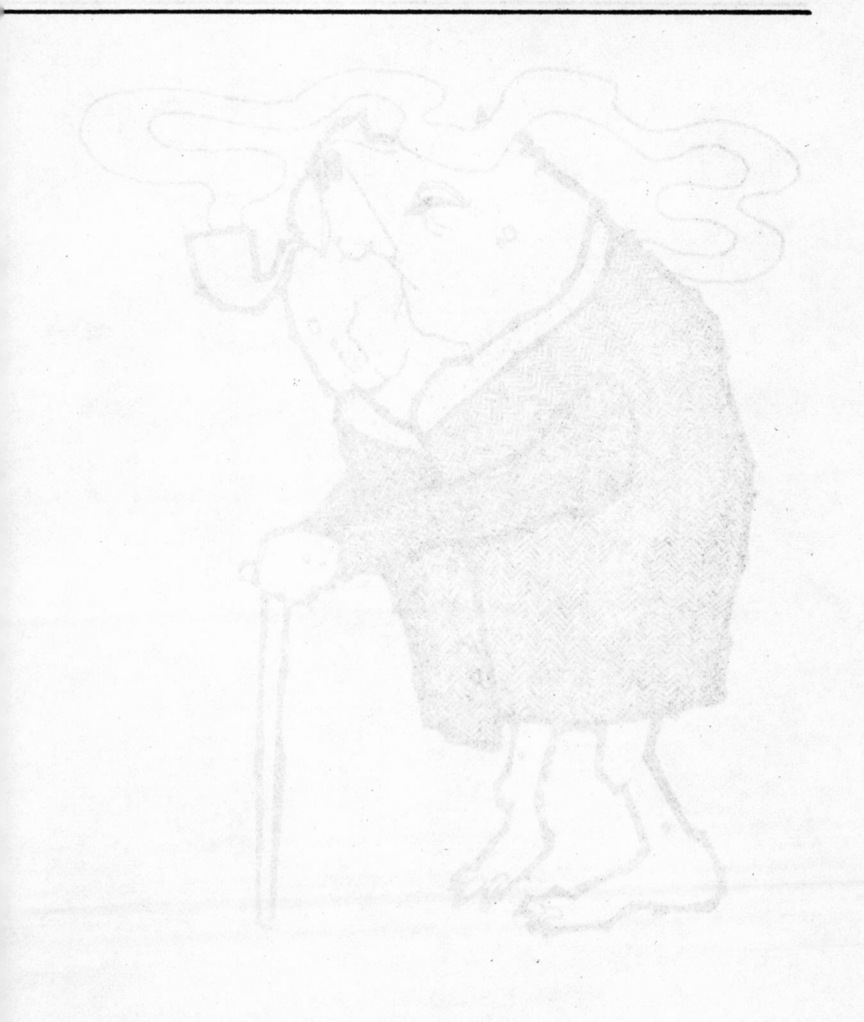

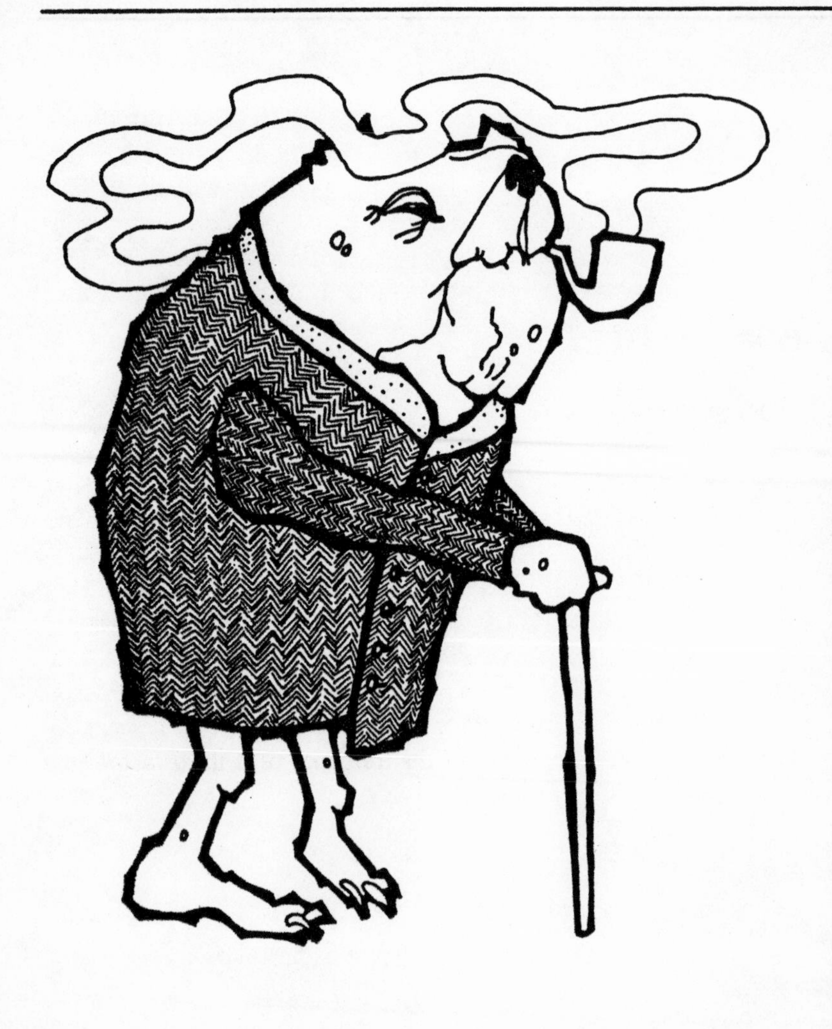

1. Grand Confounder

The Grand Confounder is the patriarch of them all. He's the original deceiver, that Grand Old Goblin of wrong conclusions, that fatal flaw every researcher would like to ban from the premises. But no matter how we bolt the doors and bar the windows, we can never be absolutely sure that when we turn around we will not find the Confounder, with a gleam in his eye, blowing smoke in our faces.

DEFINITION

What looks like a causal relationship between a supposed hazard and a disease may be due to another factor not taken into consideration. This additional factor is called a *confounder*, something that confuses the correct interpretation of data. The confounding factor acts by being associated with both the hazard and the disease in a way that makes the hazard and the disease seem to be related. This situation is also known as a secondary association: the observed association between two conditions is actually secondary to the influence of a third factor (the confounding variable).

CASE STUDIES
The Gambler's Risk

In his controversial treatise, "Gambling Causes Cancer!" Dr. Al Betzerov describes findings from a large cohort study. A random sample of persons from a state in which gambling is legal was compared to a sample of persons from a neighboring, nongambling state. Subjects were matched by age, sex, urban or rural residence, and family income. These two groups were followed for ten years, by which time a marked excess of cancer deaths had occurred among persons exposed to legalized gambling. Using these data, Dr. Betzerov estimated that 86,000 cancer deaths a year could be prevented by the prohibition of commercial gambling. Furthermore, Dr. Betzerov projected that additional thousands of senseless deaths could be averted by outlawing bingo parlors, football pools, and penny-pitching.

Comment

The problem with Dr. Betzerov's study is not what he measured, but what he did not measure. The adjacent states he chose for his study were Nevada and Utah. Although these two states are very similar in the average income of residents, number of physicians, and so forth, they differ in one important aspect. The residents of Utah are predominantly Mormons, while those in Nevada are not. Mormons differ from the general population in a number of life-style factors, including abstention from caffeine, tobacco, and alcohol. The contribution of tobacco smoke alone to cancer mortality would be enough to cause a difference in cancer deaths between the two groups. Dr. Betzerov's failure to take other factors into consideration confounded his findings. The supposed association between gambling and cancer was actually secondary to the effect of smoking, alcohol, and other factors, which acted as confounding variables (Fig. 1).

Problems of confounding are a major source of controversy in epidemiologic research. The following true examples give an idea of the extent of this problem.

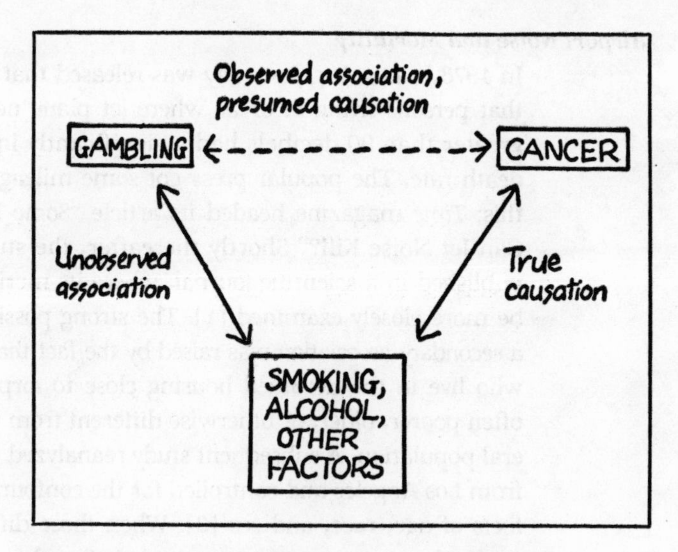

Figure 1. Association between gambling and cancer, confounded by smoking, alcohol, and other factors.

Airport Noise and Mortality

In 1978, a Los Angeles study was released that showed that persons living in areas where jet plane noise was greater than 90 decibels had a significantly increased death rate. The popular press got some mileage out of this: *Time* magazine headed its article "Sonic Doom—Can Jet Noise Kill?" Shortly thereafter, the study was published in a scientific journal, where its merits could be more closely examined [1]. The strong possibility of a secondary association was raised by the fact that people who live in the devalued housing close to airports are often poorer, older, or otherwise different from the general population. A subsequent study reanalyzed the data from Los Angeles and controlled for the confounding effects of age, race, and sex [2]. When those differences were taken into account, jet noise was found to have no effect on mortality.

Altitude and Heart Attacks

In 1977, researchers reported a decline in coronary heart disease mortality associated with higher elevations of residence in New Mexico [3]. Various possible confounders were considered but dismissed; these included white-nonwhite differences, smoking habits, and hardness of water. The authors concluded that living at higher altitude provided some protection from death due to heart disease.

Two years later, another group of researchers presented additional data from New Mexico in which "whites" were separated into Hispanic and Anglo [4]. According to these authors, some of the apparent protection conferred by altitude actually reflected different rates of disease between Anglos and Hispanics. Hispanics have lower rates of heart disease mortality than Anglos, and also tend to live in counties with higher altitudes. Thus, the authors proposed that the earlier finding of an association between altitude and mortality was a secondary association due to inadequate consideration of ethnic group as a confounder. The original authors defended their findings as valid at least for Anglo men [5]. The underlying cause-and-effect relationship of altitude to heart disease remains unresolved.

Estrogens and Endometrial Cancer

There has been extended controversy over a possible secondary association in the relation of estrogen medications and endometrial cancer. Several studies using the case-control design have shown a strong relation between endometrial cancer and the prior use of estrogens to control symptoms of menopause [6–10]. These observations have been dismissed as secondary association by other researchers [11] who propose the following. A side effect of estrogen use is uterine bleeding, which is also a symptom of endometrial cancer. Women using estrogens may be more likely to be referred for diagnostic tests for endometrial cancer. Thus, women using estrogens would be over-represented among women with endometrial cancer, creating an apparent (but secondary) association between estrogen use and cancer. While the weight of evidence supports a carcinogenic role for estrogens, the possible extent of confounding continues to be debated.

Antibiotics and Infectious Disease

Certainly no association could be less controversial than the rapid decline of infectious diseases following the advent of immunization and antibiotics. Or could it? Even so plausible a relation as this has been accused of being at least partly confounded. In his book, *The Role of Medicine: Dream, Mirage or Nemesis?* McKeown [12] presents data showing that the decline in the incidence of common infectious diseases began at the turn of this century, prior to the development of immunizations and antibiotics. He suggests that this decline was due to improving hygiene and nutrition. The introduction of specific anti-infectious therapies came, in most cases, after the incidences of infectious disease had already declined 75 percent or more from levels in the mid-1800s. McKeown proposes that some of the decline in infectious diseases even subsequent to immunizations and antibiotics is properly attributed to a continuation of the effects of improved living conditions. While his conclusions may be controversial, the point is well taken. Where the Grand Confounder is concerned, no finding is sacred.

The threat of possible confounding is a fundamental concern in all studies of human health. Many of the beasts described in the following chapters have their effect through confounding: Ecologic Fallacy, Selection Bias, Berkson Bias, and Hawthorne Effect are all variants or special examples of confounding. Given the importance of the Grand Confounder, numerous methodologic and analytic approaches have been developed to trap him. But you can make a good start in dealing with confounding by using one simple tool. Ask yourself, "Is there some plausible explanation for this finding besides direct cause and effect?"

REFERENCES

1. Meecham, W. C., and Shaw, N. Effects of jet noise on mortality rates. *Br. J. Audiol.* 13:77, 1979.
2. Frerichs, R. R., Beeman, B. L., and Coulson, A. H. Los Angeles airport noise and mortality—Faulty analysis and public policy. *Am. J. Public Health* 70:357, 1980.
3. Mortimer, E. A., Monson, R. R., and MacMahon, B. Reduction in mortality from coronary heart disease in men residing at high altitude. *N. Engl. J. Med.* 296:581, 1977.
4. Buechley, B. W., Key, C. R., Morris, D. L., et al. Altitude and ischemic heart disease in tricultural New Mexico: An example of confounding. *Am. J. Epidemiol.* 109:663, 1979.
5. Mortimer, E. A., Monson, R. R., and MacMahon, B. Comment on "Altitude and ischemic heart disease in tri-cultural New Mexico: An example of confounding." *Am. J. Epidemiol.* 109:719, 1979.

6. Smith, D. C., Prentice, R., Thompson, D. J., et al. Association of exogenous estrogens and endometrial carcinoma. *N. Engl. J. Med.* 293:1164, 1975.
7. Ziel, H. K., Finkle, W. D. Increased risk of endometrial carcinoma among users of conjugated estrogens. *N. Engl. J. Med.* 293:1167, 1975.
8. Mack, T. M., Pike, M. C., Henderson, B. E., et al. Estrogens and endometrial cancer in a retirement community. *N. Engl. J. Med.* 294:1262, 1976.
9. McDonald, T. W., Annegers, J. F., O'Fallon, W. M., et al. Exogenous estrogen and endometrial carcinoma: Case-control and incidence study. *Am J. Obstet. Gynecol.* 127:572, 1977.
10. Gray, L. A., Christopherson, W. M., Hoover, R. N. Estrogens and endometrial carcinoma. *Obstet. Gynecol.* 49:385, 1977.
11. Horwitz, R. I., Feinstein, A. R. Alternative analytic methods for case-control studies of estrogens and endometrial cancer. *N. Engl. J. Med.* 299:1089, 1978.
12. McKeown, T. *The Role of Medicine: Dream, Mirage or Nemesis?* London: Nuffield Provincial Hospitals Trust, 1976.

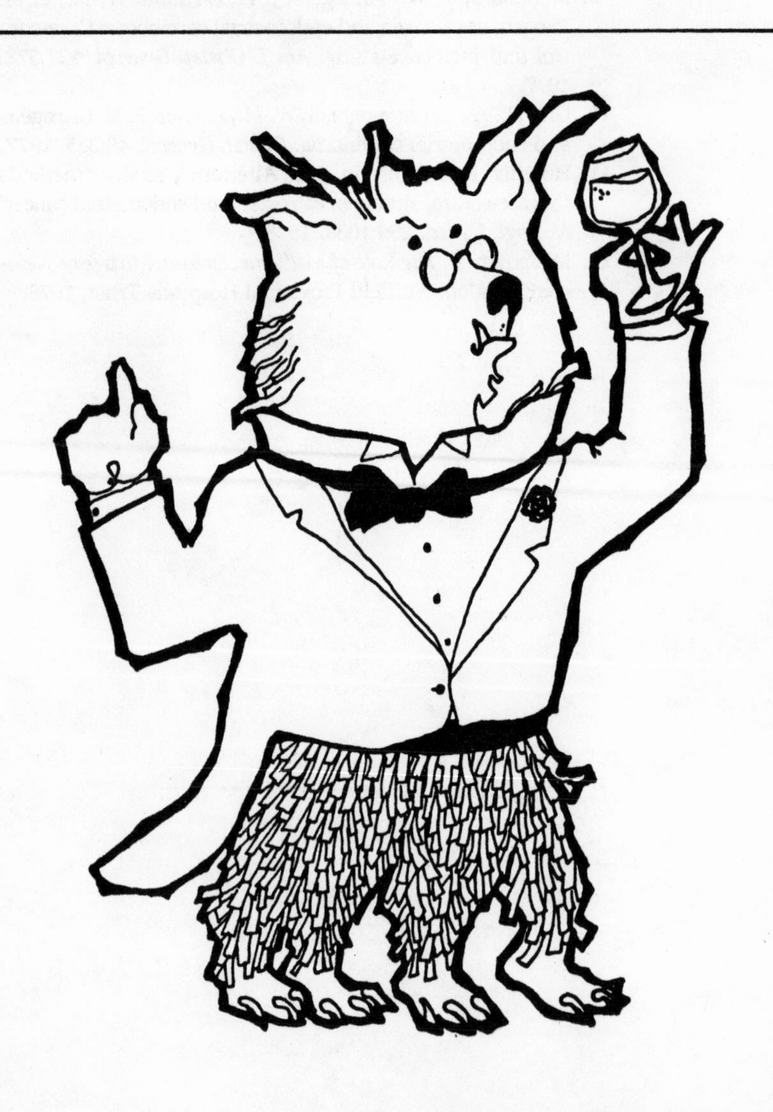

2. Numerator Monster

And there, rising from his chair at the Club, is the Numerator Monster, elegant, suave, and impeccably self-confident. The Numerator Monster elevates skimpy data to the level of Truth; he succeeds because he appears so respectable. After all, he is descended from a long lineage of revered Case Reports. Aided by his pedigree, Numerator Monster is all dignity and aplomb, with an air of utter conviction. His pronouncements are delivered with gravity and, too often, received with reverence. His failing, alas, is that he draws all his fascinating associations from within his own coterie (a cluster of cases) without regard to the population from which the cases come.

DEFINITION

Numerator data are information about the health of persons without reference to the population from which those persons come. More specifically, numerator data are half of the information needed to calculate a disease rate. A disease rate consists of the number of persons with a particular condition, divided by the total number of persons at risk. Disease rates are a fundamental tool of the epidemiologist for describing characteristics of diseases.

CASE STUDIES

The Hard Sell

A medical journal carries a full-color, two-page advertisement for a combination tranquilizer and mood elevator. On the first page is a photograph of a gentleman who could be anybody's uncle. His irritable bowel syndrome is causing him discomfort and embarrassment. Accompanying his picture is the following story.

A. B. is a 63-year-old male with a several year history of episodic borborygmi, cramps, flatulence, and diarrhea. Previous workups for intestinal parasites, allergies, and inflammatory bowel disease have been negative. Efforts to regulate diet have not affected his symptoms. Upon examination, the patient showed signs of mild depression and anxiety. A therapeutic course of Serenital was accompanied by progressive relief of symptoms. The patient has successfully returned to his Tuesday night bowling league.

On the second page is the word SERENITAL in two-inch letters and a photograph of bowling pins fanned out in a strike.

The Duck Deformity

Dr. Hugh Dewey of St. Louis observed in his obstetrics practice a number of newborn infants with webbed toes. Shortly thereafter he discovered a report of an association of citrus peel ingestion with webbing of the toes among laboratory rats. Prompted by these data, he did a nutritional survey of the mothers of these children in his practice and dashed off the following letter to the editor of a well-known medical journal.

To the Editor: Several common citrus fruits contain in their rind chemicals that a laboratory study has found to be teratogenic. The particular defect is webbed toes ("duckfoot") and, more rarely, a *cri du canard*. However, there has been no report of this finding in humans.

In the past eighteen months I have seen three infants with

webbing of the toes born to mothers who ingested orange peel during pregnancy. None of these mothers was exposed to other known teratogens, and none of the other family members was reported to have webbing. Although the exact dates of ingestion could not be determined, all episodes occurred within the early weeks of gestation.

These clinical and experimental data suggest that citrus rind causes birth defects. It is recommended that pregnant women abstain from orange peel and food products containing citrus rind.

Comment

Numerator data, if nothing else, are usually interesting. These data describe people who have gotten sick or who have gotten well, presumably because of some associated event. The challenge is to give only as much weight to this information as it deserves. Numerator data are a statement of reasonable hypothesis, illustrated by an example of an association that may or may not be coincidence.

Case reports are a respectable and ritualized form of numerator data with a long tradition in medical literature. The astute observation of a few cases can be the first step toward discovery of a genuine cause-and-effect relationship. In a few notable instances, the report of numerator data alone has been a scientific landmark. For example, the discovery that maternal rubella could cause birth defects was made by an Australian ophthalmologist who noted an outbreak of congenital cataracts in conjunction with an epidemic of German measles [1]. More often, numerator data are merely the beginning of an extended process of investigation. Many times, numerator data are not supported by subsequent studies, and the hypothesis is discarded. In any event, numerator data alone are seldom sufficient to establish a causal relation.

Consider the first case. The journal advertisement bases its claim of efficacy on a single concrete example. If this success story had come from a medical colleague, many clinicians might be persuaded to consider trying this new therapy. Shouldn't the pharmaceutical company be allowed the same consideration? Surely there is no error of fact in the advertisement. But, you might ask yourself, what is the denominator? This example was a success, but out of how many attempts?

In contrast to the average clinician, a manufacturer is required to compile large quantities of clinical data concerning the effectiveness of its drugs. The manufacturer in this case selected one successful case report out of many therapeutic attempts. For all we know, this case might have been the *only* success. Such is the device of the Numerator Monster. Like so many of the beasts, the Numerator Monster deludes with half-truths. Although this advertisement was fictitious, real-life examples of this form of persuasion abound [2].

Dr. Dewey's problem with birth defects and the Numerator Monster is more subtle. He has observed three cases of webbed toes associated with exposure to orange peel. The occurrence of any new or unusual exposure in association with a disease is often the basis for a case report. Such observations are especially compelling when accompanied by corroborative experimental data, as was true in this example. However, case reports may also be deceptive, as Dr. Dewey learned to his dismay.

Shortly after publication of his report, a colleague wrote to him to point out that a current nutritional fad among pregnant women included the use of citrus rind for low-calorie flavoring. Had Dr. Dewey interviewed mothers of *normal* infants to determine if they also had been eating orange rind? He had not, and when he did, Dr. Dewey found that practically everyone in his practice was consuming orange rind during pregnancy. He braced himself for an epidemic of webbed toes, but as luck would have it, none occurred. The original observation of three babies with webbing had been a chance occurrence.

Dr. Dewey deserves credit for his alertness. He pursued

a hunch that might have led to the discovery of a new teratogen. Fortunately, his recommendation that pregnant women abstain from orange peels did no harm, even if it did no good. In other situations, however, case reports may prompt actions that are unnecessarily alarming or costly.

Consider a recent letter in the pages of *The Lancet* [3]. The authors reported that of seven children with childhood bone marrow failure, all had been exposed to pesticides. The pesticides contained chemicals that cause leukemia in laboratory animals. While an association between pesticide exposure and bone marrow failure is plausible, this finding deserves to be interpreted with caution. This report came from a military base, where crowded quarters and high resident turnover may lead to frequent use of roach or ant sprays. It is possible that *any* person on the base whom these authors chose to study would report exposure to insecticides. This possibility can be explored in several ways. The easiest question to ask would be, do children with bone marrow failure really differ in their exposure to pesticides from other children living on the base? This would, in effect, be a case control approach. More fundamentally, what is the denominator for the authors' finding? In other words, what is the total number of children on the base, and what proportion is exposed to pesticides? Is the occurrence of marrow failure higher in their population than would be expected in the general population? A study that asked these latter questions would be using a cohort design.

Questions like these do not invalidate a case report. They *do* emphasize that numerator data are usually not persuasive evidence by themselves. To guard against overinterpreting numerator data, ask yourself, "What is the denominator? What is the total population at risk? Is the rate of occurrence really different than expected?"

If the denominator is unknown, be cautious. The Numerator Monster may be luring you out on a limb.

REFERENCES

1. Gregg, N. M. Congenital cataract following German measles in the mother. *Trans. Ophthalmol. Soc. Aust.* 3:35, 1941.
2. Advertisement. *N. Engl. J. Med.* 298:lvi, 1978.
3. Reeves, J. D., Driggers, D. A., and Kiley, V. A. Household insecticide–associated aplastic anemia and acute leukemia in children (letter). *The Lancet* II:300, 1981.

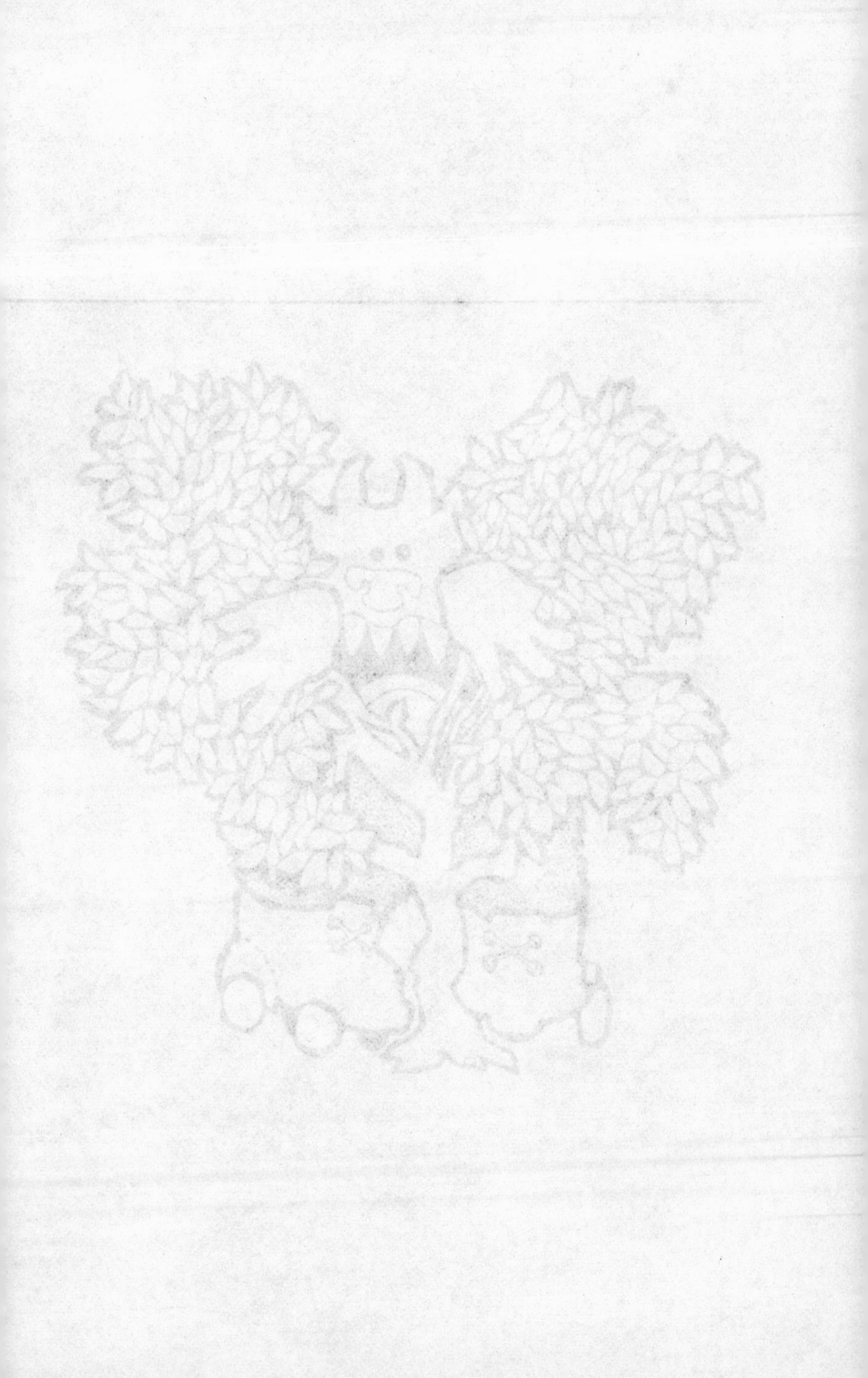

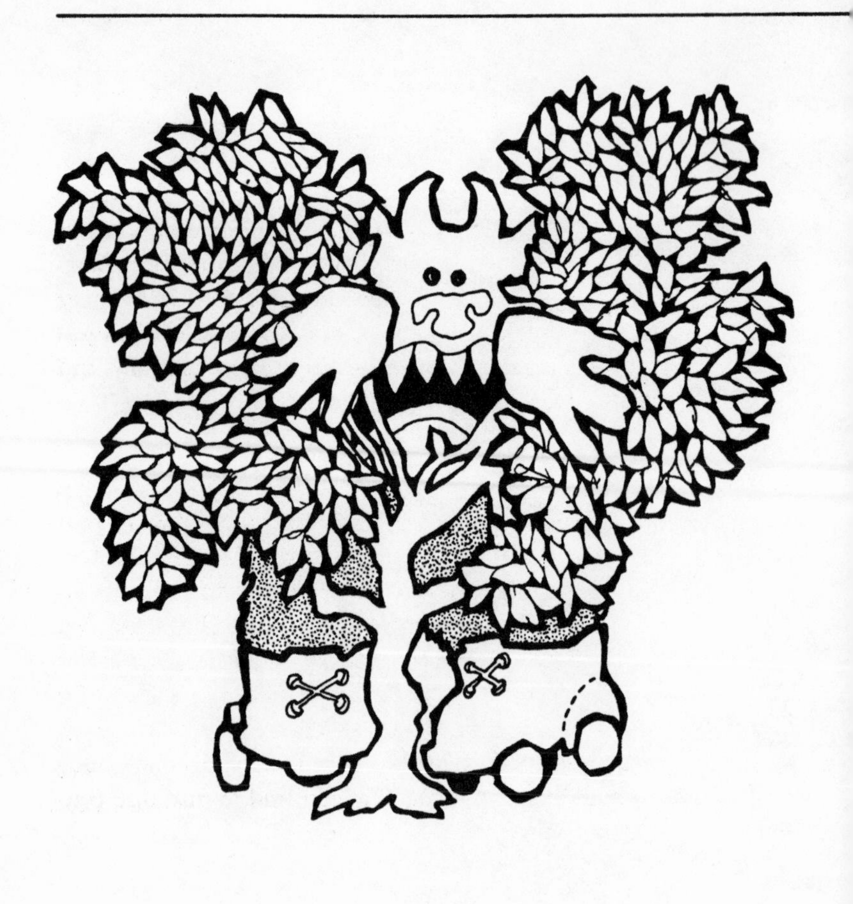

3. Selection Bias

The Selection Bias is a sneaky beast with a hardy constitution. Although he is one of the most common beasts in medical research, he is seldom sighted in the open. Instead, he lurks in the shallow underbrush at the fringes of unsuspecting research projects. Sometimes he snatches away particular study subjects before the researcher arrives. Other times he steals subjects right out from under the researcher's nose. The only way to protect one's self from this beast is to choose study subjects carefully, and then to guard them with vigilance.

DEFINITION

Persons being studied may differ in important ways from the larger population they are claimed to represent or from a second group of persons with whom they are supposedly comparable. The reason for such differences often lies in the way persons become study subjects. Certain people may be more likely than others to be selected for a study or to stay in a study—often for reasons unknown to the researcher. When selective factors make the study group different in a way that can lead to mistaken conclusions, selection bias has occurred.

CASE STUDY
Labor Complications in Bearclaw

Dr. U. Kahn is the newest partner in an obstetrics practice in Bearclaw, Alaska. During her first year, she noticed that complications of labor seemed to be more common in winter months. She decided to collect data on the length of labor and the number of labor complications by reviewing hospital records from the previous two years. Dr. Kahn found that the hospital data confirmed her impressions (Table 1). The mean duration of labor was 2½ hours longer in winter months than in summer months ($p<.01$). The incidence of labor complications went up from 7.8% to 11.7% in the winter months ($p=.04$).

Dr. Kahn speculated that the seasonal decline in ultraviolet radiation interacted with local seasonal dietary changes to disrupt fetal adrenal function and thus complicate the course of labor. The next step seemed obvious. It was time for a clinical trial of sunlamps and multivitamins for women due to deliver in winter months to see if the winter increase in complications could be prevented.

Just as Dr. Kahn was about to order a crate of sunlamps, it occurred to her that there might be a beast in her data. Selection bias occurs when a group of study subjects differs in some important way from another group it supposedly resembles. In this case, Dr. Kahn had assumed that women who came to the hospital in winter months were no different from women who came in summer. However, she was also aware that some women who came for prenatal care ended up delivering their babies at home, especially if labor seemed to be progressing smoothly. When she discussed this with one of her partners, he pointed out that home deliveries were much more common in winter, when travel conditions were poor. Women who would come to the hospital for a delivery in the summer might be more likely to stay home in the

Table 1. Duration of labor and occurrence of labor complications among hospital deliveries in Bearclaw, Alaska

Season	Hospital deliveries	Mean duration of labor	Labor complications
Summer (4 months)	180	8.0 hr	7.8% (14/180)
Winter (8 months)	240	10.5 hr*	11.7%** (28/240)

*$p < .01$
**$p = .04$

Table 2. Duration of labor and occurrence of labor complications among hospital *and* home deliveries in Bearclaw, Alaska

Season	Hospital deliveries	Home deliveries	All deliveries	Mean duration of labor	Labor complications
Summer	180	20	200	8.0 hr	8.0% (16/200)
Winter	240	160	400	8.0 hr	8.0% (32/400)

winter, especially if labor was rapid. On the other hand, women with prolonged or complicated labor would make every attempt to reach the hospital regardless of the season.

Dr. Kahn went back to the clinic files to find the records of women who had delivered at home. In fact, home deliveries were much more common in winter. Furthermore, the rate of labor complications among home deliveries was very low. This reflected the selective tendency of women with normal labors to stay home. When Dr. Kahn added these home deliveries to her data, the higher risk of winter deliveries disappeared (Table 2). The seasonal trend in complications had been an artifact of the selective removal of normal deliveries from the hospital-delivered group during winter months.

Comment

Selection bias can take many forms. For instance, selection bias can exaggerate the apparent severity of diseases. Persons who seek medical attention for a disease are likely to be those who are the sickest with that disease. This leads the physician to conclude that the disease is more debilitating than it actually is [1]. One example is cytomegalovirus infection. Because the first persons in whom the disease was diagnosed were those with severe disease, this virus was initially thought to be highly virulent. As more people were tested for the virus, it became clear that the virus is widespread and only rarely leads to serious illness.

Another form of selection bias can occur before a study even begins. Persons who move from one city or state to another may do so for reasons related to their health. For example, people with chronic lung disease may move away from polluted industrial towns in favor of more pastoral areas. Such selective migration could lead to a higher concentration of persons with lung disease in pollution-free areas than in industrial towns. A subsequent study of the geographic distribution of lung disease might result in the erroneous conclusion that living in low-pollution areas is more likely to cause disease than living in high-pollution areas.

A major opportunity for selection bias occurs when a large proportion of the original study population is never actually studied. Some loss of study subjects is to be expected in any study. However, the larger the proportion of persons lost or excluded, the larger the possibility that those included are a biased sample.

Selection bias can intervene even after study subjects have been enlisted in the research project. It is a rare study that doesn't lose some subjects along the way. People quit, die, or move away. It is very likely that the persons who are lost will differ in important ways from those who remain. As a general rule, the more subjects who are lost, the less useful are the results from the remainder. Whenever possible, the researcher should compare the study subjects to the drop-outs or other lost persons to estimate whether the two groups might differ in a way that could bias the results.

There are some investigators so reckless as to deliberately exclude, substitute, or add cases after a study is in progress. This is an open invitation to Selection Bias. The beast seldom passes up this opportunity to do his mischief.

EXAMPLES

Ellenberg, J.H., and Nelson, K. B. Sample selection and the natural history of disease: Studies of febrile seizures. *J.A.M.A.* 243:1337, 1980.

The authors review studies of childhood febrile seizures and find that population-based studies consistently report low rates of unfavorable sequelae, while clinic-based studies report higher and more variable rates of unfavorable sequelae. The authors conclude that when subjects are drawn from a clinic population selection bias contributes to a distorted description of the natural history of this disease.

Seltzer, C. C., and Jablon, S. Effects of selection on mortality. *Am. J. Epidemiol.* 100:376, 1974.

The authors demonstrate that, as a result of the screening process by which they are chosen, United States Army inductees are a very nonrepresentative group of persons. Since only the healthy are inducted, their risk of disease both while in the army and after discharge is less than that for the general population. This effect lingers for years after discharge. As a result, any study of army veterans that compares their health status to the general population's health status must reckon with the selection bias involved.

SUGGESTED READING

Kleinbaum, D. G., Morganstern, H., and Kupper, L. L. Selection bias in epidemiologic studies. *Am. J. Epidemiol.* 113:452, 1981.

REFERENCE

1. Motulsky, A. G. Biased ascertainment and the natural history of diseases. *N. Engl. J. Med.* 298:1196, 1978.

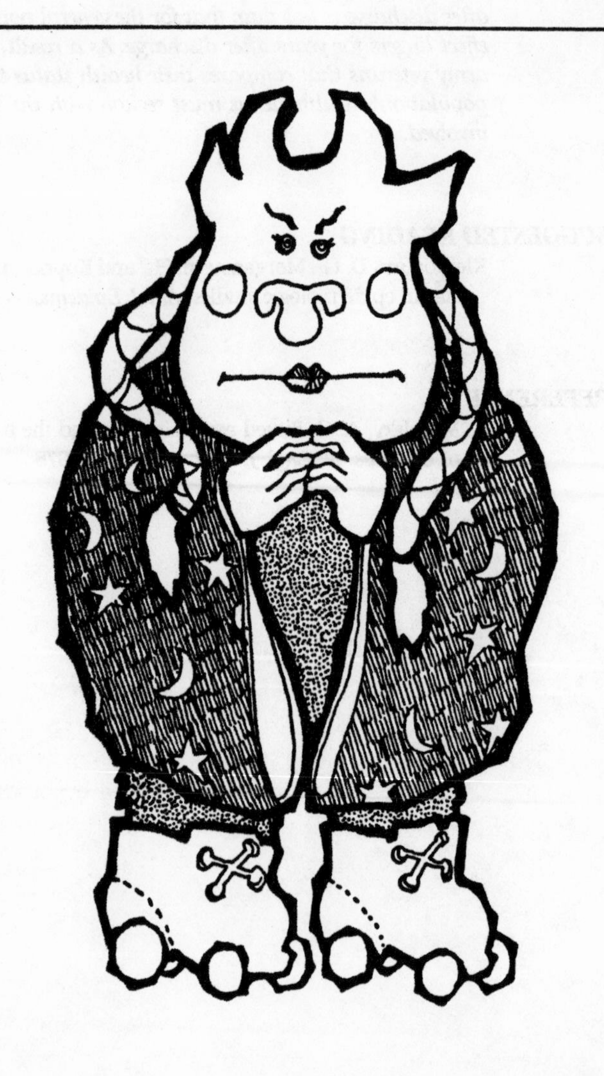

4. Response Bias

Response Bias is one of the more insidious creatures you are likely to encounter in your journeys through the medical literature. She will systematically undermine a research protocol by luring subjects into forgetfulness and inaccuracy—deliberate and unintentional. Pigtailed and cloaked in innocence, she insinuates herself into even the most sophisticated research designs. Her trick is always the same: she mysteriously influences how people respond to an investigator's questions so that their answers are distorted. The wary researcher (and the alert reader) must be particularly careful to watch for the veiled bias of this siren on skates.

DEFINITION

Response bias is the systematic error that results when subjects respond inaccurately to an investigator's questions. *How* people answer a questionnaire is the salient feature of this form of bias, since people's reports of events, symptoms, personal characteristics, or habits are often crucial to the proper study of a hypothesis. Response bias is distinguished from selection bias, which is a systematic error related to *whether* subjects respond.

CASE STUDY
The Impaired Physician in Lushton County

Over the past several years, widespread interest has focused on the impaired physician—the doctor whose medical judgments or abilities are altered by the use of alcohol or drugs. The national news media have been quick to capitalize on the public interest generated by such physicians, and some surveys suggest that as many as 10 percent of practicing physicians are impaired sufficiently to endanger the health of their patients.

The Lushton County Medical Society, like many other medical societies around the country, had received a number of inquiries about the problem of impaired physicians. Most of the callers simply wanted to know if Lushton had a problem, although a few people complained about certain physicians.

Concerned by the growing number of inquiries, Dr. Brunus Beefsteak, president of the Lushton County Medical Society, commissioned a survey of community perceptions regarding physician impairment. One thousand persons were randomly chosen from the community and sent a simple postcard. Persons were asked for anonymous impressions regarding their personal physician. In particular, the survey requested the patients' perceptions regarding drug- or alcohol-related impairment of *their* physician's practice of medicine. Additionally, patients were asked to estimate the degree of impairment among all physicians in Lushton County.

Dr. Beefsteak's results are shown in Table 3. Ninety-eight percent of the study sample had returned their cards. Fewer than one percent of the respondents felt that their own physician's judgment was impaired because of drug or alcohol abuse, but nearly 80 percent reported that they believed the professional image of Lushton County physicians had been tarnished by doctors' drug or alcohol abuse. Furthermore, 85 percent felt that physicians who use drugs or alcohol are a threat to their patients.

Table 3. Impaired physician survey

Question	Positive response (%)
1. Is *your* physician's medical judgment ever compromised by the use of alcohol or drugs?	0.4
2. Does physician drug or alcohol abuse threaten the professional image of physicians in Lushton?	78
3. Are physicians who use drugs or alcohol a threat to their patients?	85

Beefsteak interpreted these results to mean that Lushton physicians are almost universally viewed as unimpaired by the patients who know them well. However, the news media had successfully tainted the image of doctors through a biased campaign of critical sensationalism. Pleased with the survey results, the medical society executive board sent copies to the local newspapers in the hope of stemming the recent adverse publicity with carefully gathered, objective information.

Comment

The *State Medical News* ran the following story on Dr. Beefsteak's study.

The Lushton County Medical Society just completed a survey of nearly 1,000 patients regarding drug and alcohol use by their personal physicians. Fewer than one percent of patients felt that their physician's judgment was jeopardized or altered by the use of drugs or alcohol. These patients were, however, aware of the problem since 80 percent agreed that physician drug or alcohol abuse is a potential threat to patients. In these days of widespread debauchery and immorality, it is comforting to learn that the medical community has remained a bastion of upright and high-minded behavior.

The community of Lushton accepted the results of this study until the state attorney general cited 42 Lushton physicians for drug- or alcohol-related malpractice during the previous three years. This amounted to 12 percent of licensed physicians in the county. Thus, while a sizable number of the county's physicians had records showing substance abuse problems, fewer than one percent of the Lushton patient sample felt their physicians were ever compromised by drugs or alcohol. Dr. Beefsteak's survey was inconsistent with the actual record of physician performance. Why was the study so inaccurate? Because the credibility of the Lushton County Medical Society was in jeopardy, a follow-up study was commissioned.

Ten percent of the original 1,000 respondents were

Table 4. Follow-up survey results

Question	Positive response (%)
1. Is *your* physician's medical judgment ever compromised by the use of alcohol or drugs?	8
2. Does physician drug or alcohol abuse threaten the professional image of physicians in Lushton?	80
3. Are physicians who use drugs or alcohol a threat to their patients?	82

selected for home interviews. They were first assured confidentiality and then asked detailed questions about their physician's performance. Much to the executive committee's surprise, the results this time were quite different.

As indicated in Table 4, eight percent of the patients now felt their physician's judgment was at one time or another compromised by alcohol or drugs. When asked why they had changed their answers this time, most people said they had been reluctant to criticize their own physicians. They did not, however, hesitate to criticize the profession as a whole: 80 percent stated again that drug and alcohol abuse threatened the image of Lushton physicians. With this better understanding of the extent of the problem, the medical society has put major emphasis on identifying and counseling the impaired physicians.

Any investigation like Dr. Beefsteak's that relies on accurate responses to a questionnaire can fall prey to the talents of Response Bias. There are many things besides a reluctance to criticize that can affect the way people answer questionnaires. People with a disease may tend to recall events, drug exposures, and the like differently than those not so affected. The same is true for families and friends of persons who have died or parents of babies with birth defects. These people are more likely to have examined past experiences for explanations of recent events, and thus may be more likely to report things that other people would forget. Questionnaire design and interviewer-respondent interaction can also affect how a person remembers and answers.

We, as readers, must always remember the effects Response Bias can have on the results and conclusions of a study. If the authors acknowledge her possible presence in their discussion of methods or results, we are inclined to feel more confident about the conclusions.

EXAMPLES

Adatto, K., Doebele, K. G., Galland, L., and Grandewetter, L. Behavioral factors and urinary tract infection. *J.A.M.A.* 241:2525, 1979.

Women with recurrent urinary tract infections report urinary hesitancy more often than matched controls. Is it possible that women with recurrent infections are more conscious of their urinary habits and thus more likely to remember delayed micturition than other women?

Kilbourne, E. M., Choi, K., Jones, S., Thacher, S. B., and The Field Investigation Team. Risk factors for heat stroke. A case-control study. *J.A.M.A.* 247:3332, 1982.

This study details the risk factors for heat stroke as determined by interviews with a close friend or family member of patients who died, with surviving patients, and with matched controls. Survivors and family members of patients who died may be more likely to recall previous conditions, medications, and recent activities than the controls. This response bias could affect the conclusions of the study.

Waldman, R. J., Hall, W. M., McGee, H., and VonAmburg, G. Aspirin as a risk factor in Reye's Syndrome. *J.A.M.A.* 247:3089, 1982.

In order to reduce the effects of response bias, interviews with patients and controls were conducted soon after identification of an index case. Recall of important information surrounding the time of the illness was controlled as much as possible by interviewing cases and controls at similar times in the course of a viral illness. By acknowledging the potential for such bias the authors enhance confidence in the results.

Zeiss, C. R., Wolkonsky, P., Chason, R., et al. Syndromes in workers exposed to trimellitic anhydride. *Ann. Intern. Med.* 98:9, 1983.

All workers in a factory exposed to the industrial chemical trimellitic anhydride were enrolled in a longitudinal study of allergic phenomena. Because the researchers were not blinded to the exposure status of the worker, they may have questioned the workers with known exposure more closely.

SUGGESTED READING

Feinstein, A. R. Clinical biostatistics. XVIII. Efficacy of different research structures in preventing bias in the analysis of causation. *Clin. Pharmacol. Ther.* 26:129, 1979.

A general review of several types of bias including response bias.

Hayden, G. F., Kramer, M. S., and Horwitz, R. I. The case-control study. A practical review for the clinician. *J.A.M.A.* 247:326, 1982.

Examples of studies affected by different types of bias are given. Among the studies cited where response bias may have affected the results are the observed associations between endometrial cancer and estrogens, and between measles and the risk of subacute sclerosing panencephalitis.

Jason, J., Andereck, N. D., Marks, J., and Tyler, C. W. Child abuse in Georgia: A method to evaluate risk factors and reporting bias. *Am. J. Public Health* 72:1353, 1982.

Voluntary case reporting can result in erroneous conclusions about the demography of child abuse. Other conditions that are voluntarily reported are subject to the same potential problems. This type of response bias can be reduced by an inexpensive follow-up system described in this article.

Mann, J. M. A prospective study of response error in food history questionnaires: Implications for food borne outbreak investigation. *Am. J. Public Health* 71:1362, 1981.

In a prospective study of responses from people attending a pot luck luncheon only 73 percent correctly recalled any single food item. The potential effects of response bias for investigations of food-borne disease outbreaks is discussed.

Rabkin, J. G., and Struening, E. L. Life events, stress, and illness. *Science* 194:1013, 1976.

The literature on life events and illness is riddled with the confusing effects of response bias after a major illness. The authors discuss how this affects any conclusions we may draw from this body of literature.

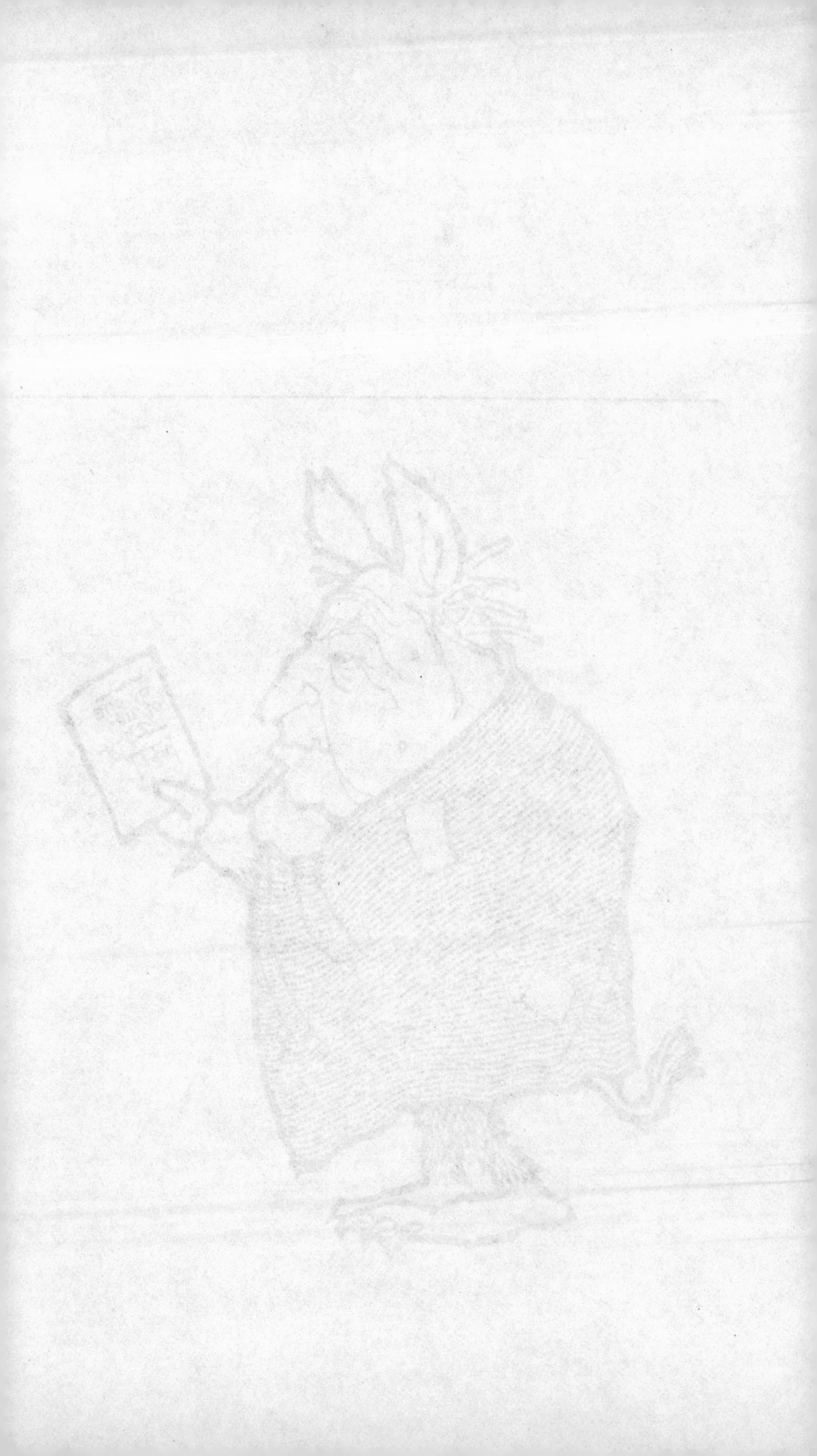

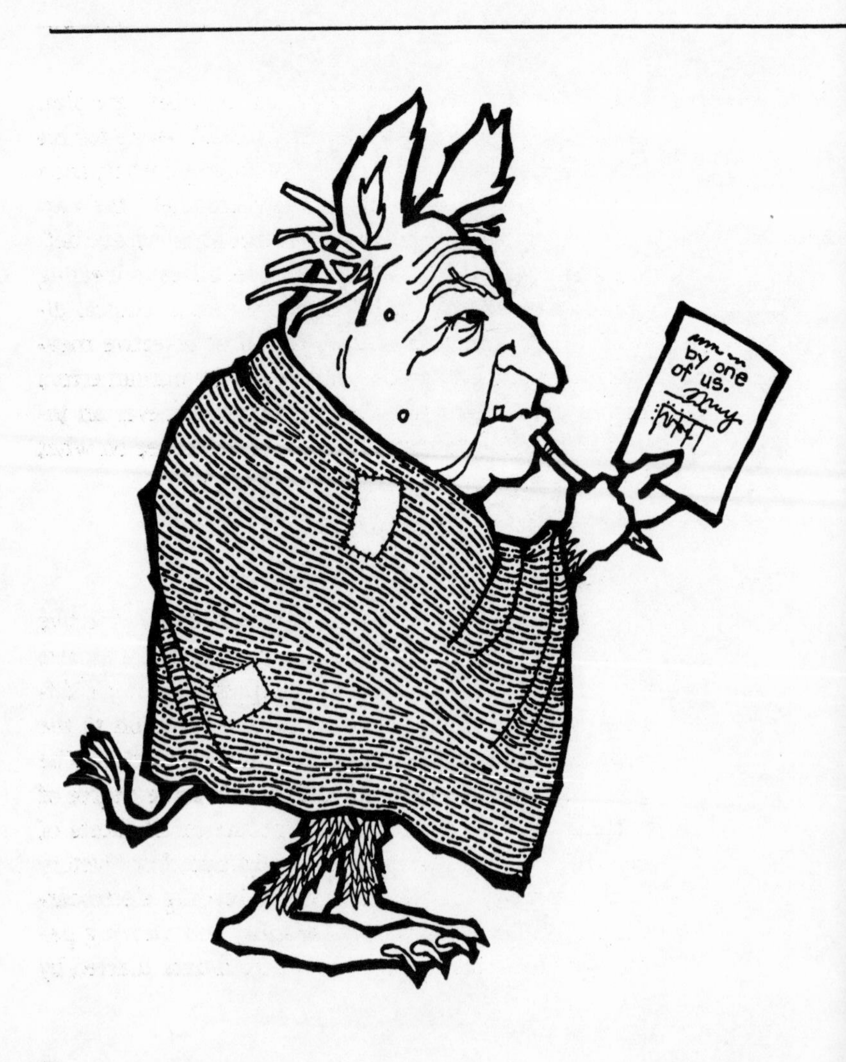
by one
of us.

5. Variable Observer

The Variable Observer is a seasoned, crotchety gremlin. He is widely esteemed among biomedical beasts for his years of clinical experience and his willing participation in all forms of clinical research. Unfortunately, the Variable Observer tends to apply his rather idiosyncratic definitions to investigational work. He specializes in creating faulty conclusions through inconsistencies in clinical diagnosis and assessment. Even the most objective measurements and evaluations fall prey to the human errors he promotes. His handiwork abounds whenever an investigator assumes that all observers will agree on what they see, hear, or feel.

DEFINITION

Even when different investigators use identical objective criteria for clinical assessments important discrepancies can occur. Each observer will interpret the criteria differently and apply this individual interpretation to the collection and evaluation of clinical information. The most objective of measurements contain some degree of subjectivity. Observer variability occurs in all facets of clinical medicine and clinical investigation, from history taking and physical examination to reading electrocardiograms, interpreting radiographs, and viewing pathology slides. Conclusions drawn from data marred by

unrecognized observer variability can be skewed or downright wrong.

CASE STUDY
Megacide in the Treatment of Otitis Media

Drs. Rudolf Blind and Harry Azabat were asked by the state medical school to conduct a controlled trial of megacide, a new antibiotic for otitis media in children. Preliminary studies in otitis-prone stray cats had demonstrated that megacide was more effective than amoxicillin in sterilizing the feline middle ear. The Blind-Azabat pediatric practice was chosen for this trial of megacide because of its large patient enrollment and its long-standing relationship with the medical school.

All children between the ages of six months and six years presenting to the office with ear pulling or ear pain were randomly assigned to either Dr. Blind or Dr. Azabat. After examination by either doctor, children with otitis media were then placed on the antibiotic assigned to that doctor. Dr. Blind used amoxicillin, and Dr. Azabat used megacide. Fifty children were enrolled in each group, and at the end of treatment the children were evaluated for resolution of otitis media by an ear, nose, and throat specialist at the medical school.

Table 5 shows the results of this trial. Eighty percent of the children treated with megacide (Dr. Azabat) showed resolution of their otitis media, compared to 60 percent treated with amoxicillin (Dr. Blind). This difference was significant at the .05 level. The Blind-Azabat report was presented at the medical school's pediatric grand rounds and will appear in a major pediatric journal.

Pleased with the reception their work received, Drs. Blind and Azabat are seeking funding for another antibiotic study. In the meantime amoxicillin is no longer used in their practice.

Table 5. Resolution of otitis media in 100 children (study 1)

Antibiotic	Resolved (%)	Unresolved (%)
Megacide (Azabat)	40 (80)	10 (20)
Amoxicillin (Blind)	30 (60)	20 (40)

$\chi^2 = 4.76, p < .05$

Comment

A wary pediatrician from Onion Skin, Oklahoma, read the report of the megacide trial and raised the issue of observer variability. She wrote to Drs. Blind and Azabat suggesting that they repeat their study, switching the antibiotic employed by each physician. Taking up the challenge, the doctors enrolled an additional 100 children in an extension of the original study. Dr. Blind now used megacide instead of amoxicillin and Dr. Azabat used amoxicillin instead of megacide.

The results of this second trial were almost exactly opposite to the first. Of the children treated with amoxicillin by Dr. Azabat, 78 percent showed resolution, while only 58 percent treated with megacide by Dr. Blind showed resolution. It seemed Dr. Azabat was better at treating otitis media than Dr. Blind regardless of the antibiotic used!

Thoroughly confused by these results, the good doctors asked for help from the epidemiologist at the medical school. He suggested that each doctor examine the *same* patients before starting treatment and that only those children having a diagnosis of otitis media *on which they both agreed* be randomized into megacide- or amoxicillin-treated groups.

Drs. Blind and Azabat began their third study. Much to their chagrin, however, they couldn't agree on the diagnosis of otitis media in about 20 percent of the children. One hundred children on whom they did agree were finally accumulated and were randomly assigned. As in their first trial, Dr. Blind used amoxicillin and Dr. Azabat used megacide. The results are shown in Table 6. The doctors were aghast to find that the results for each antibiotic were virtually identical. They had been snared by the guile of the Variable Observer.

Where did the well-meaning pediatricians go wrong? In the first two studies the treatment results for each doctor were the same regardless of the antibiotic used.

Table 6. Resolution of otitis media in 100 children (study 3)

Antibiotic	Resolved (%)	Unresolved (%)
Megacide (Azabat)	29 (58)	21 (42)
Amoxicillin (Blind)	31 (62)	19 (38)

$\chi^2 = 0.17$, p = not significant

Table 7. The variable observer in clinical interpretation

Task (number of studies reviewed)	Range of agreement (%)
Interpret ECG (6)	21–88
Interpret chest x-rays (2)	70–78
Interpret barium enema (colitis) (1)	79–95
Interpret barium swallow (varices) (1)	81
Recognize physical signs (8)	44–97
Concur on diagnosis (4)	16–92
Assess quality of care (1)	56–84

Source: Koran [1].

When Drs. Blind and Azabat agreed upon the diagnosis before initiating treatment, their results were identical.

Dr. Azabat's better outcomes in the first two studies were due to his treating children who had less definitive signs of otitis media and would probably have had good resolution regardless of what was done. Dr. Azabat said his criteria for a diagnosis of otitis media are more liberal than Dr. Blind's. His liberal diagnosis of otitis probably led to the inclusion of milder cases in his treatment group, which made the treatment look better. The effect of the crotchety Variable Observer would have been missed if the doctors had not been alerted to the flaw in their original study design. Only then did his treachery become apparent.

The Variable Observer is common in the medical literature. Koran [1] reviewed the problem of observer variability in medicine and documented the high prevalence of nonagreement for a variety of clinical judgments. Table 7 shows the generally wide ranges of observer disagreement in the interpretation of diagnostic procedures such as electrocardiograms, chest radiographs, and liver scans. Agreement between observers ranged from 16 percent to 97 percent, depending on which diagnostic skill was tested. The reliability of any clinical observation is greatly improved if two or more people are involved in the evaluation.

Our Variable Observer preys on enthusiastic investigators who are motivated by the best of intentions. Be cautious, for most certainly when results rely on a single person's observations the Variable Observer can be found finishing up his task, ready to move on to the next study.

EXAMPLES

Baker, J. P., Detsky, A. S., Wesson, D. E., et al. Nutritional assessment. A comparison of clinical judgment and objective measurements. *N. Engl. J. Med.* 306:969, 1982.

Before comparing the two selected methods of assessing nutritional status, each patient was independently examined by two observers, each of whom determined whether nutritional status was normal, mildly abnormal, or severely abnormal. The two observers agreed in 81 percent of cases. The patients on whom there was agreement were then assessed by quantitative tests of nutritional status to check for agreement with clinical judgment. The authors thus avoided some of the problems of observer variability in the highly subjective area of global nutritional assessment.

Boerner, D. F., and Swadyk, P. The value of the sputum Gram's stain in community-acquired pneumonia. *J.A.M.A.* 247:642, 1982.

Of 45 patients with a sputum Gram's stain showing gram-positive diplococci, Streptococcus pneumoniae *grew in 29 (64%). These latter patients experienced more rapid clinical resolution than patients with either no apparent pathogen or mixed flora on Gram's stain. The importance of these results is limited by the fact that they rely on a single person's reading of the Gram's stain.*

Carter, S. A. Arterial auscultation in peripheral vascular disease. *J.A.M.A.* 246:1682, 1981.

A comparison study of arterial auscultation and quantitative measurement of peripheral arterial circulation showed a 63 percent agreement between these techniques. Since only a single observer performed the auscultation it is difficult to see how applicable these results are to other settings.

Chun, P. K. C., and Dunn, B. E. Clinical clues to severe aortic stenosis. *Arch. Intern. Med.* 142:2284, 1982.

This study compares the results of clinical assessment of the severity of aortic stenosis with results of catheterization. The authors recognize the importance of observer variability in subjective clinical assessments, but do not indicate the magnitude of variability among three observers. Without knowing the amount of variability among the clinicians or their relative expertise, it is difficult to determine if the results are generally applicable.

Lipkin, M., and Lamb, G. S. The couvade syndrome: An epidemiologic study. *Ann. Intern. Med.* 96:509, 1982.

The couvade syndrome is the occurrence of pregnancy-related symptoms (nausea, vomiting, abdominal pain) among husbands of expectant mothers. In this retrospective chart review of 300 randomly selected couples from a health maintenance organization, each mate's medical record was evaluated for symptoms consistent with a diagnosis of couvade syndrome. The authors noted that the "rating was done independently by two persons," but do not mention the percent agreement between the two observers making the diagnosis. This information would be useful to the reader evaluating the data, especially because the authors report a 25 percent prevalence of couvade syndrome.

SUGGESTED READING

Feinstein, A. R. *Clinical Judgment.* New York: Kruger, 1967. Pp.4, 90, 204–208.

This includes an excellent discussion of observer variability.

Schwartz, W. B., Wolfe, H. J., and Pauker, S. G. Pathology and probabilities. A new approach to interpreting and reporting biopsies. *N. Engl. J. Med.* 305:917, 1981.

By the application of a numerical probabilistic method to the analysis of biopsy material the authors tackle the difficult problems of observer variability among pathologists. This technique has potential use in areas such as radiology, physical examination, and diagnosis, where observer variability is a well recognized phenomenon.

Shapiro, A. R. The evaluation of clinical predictions. *N. Engl. J. Med.* 296:1509, 1977.

In this paper, a method to assess the accuracy of clinical judgments is described in detail.

REFERENCE

1. Koran, L. M. The reliability of clinical methods, data and judgments. *N. Engl. J. Med.* 293:642:695, 1975.

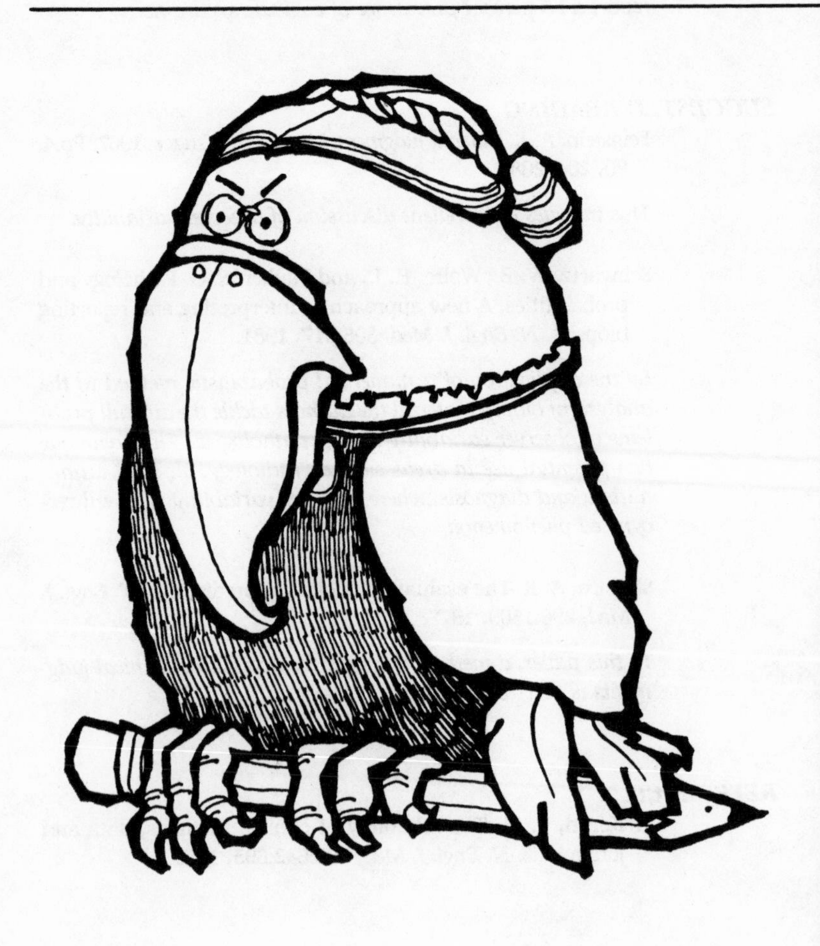

6. Hawthorne Effect

The Hawthorne Effect is the silent partner of every clinical investigator. With a deep penetrating gaze this beast makes people self-conscious of their own behavior. Her curious yet intense scrutiny is sometimes enough to cause persons to change how they act, often unconsciously. Even though her curiosity is benign, her effect can be disruptive and unpredictable. Depending on the design of the study, the Hawthorne Effect can enhance or disguise a finding. Since she is a natural part of every investigation in which people are being observed, it is impossible to keep her away. Her mere presence can influence the results of a study.

DEFINITION

The Hawthorne Effect is the epidemiologic equivalent of the uncertainty principle in physics. The act of observing a phenomenon changes the phenomenon itself. People's behavior may change just because they know they are being studied. We can never be certain that what we observe in the group under study is exactly the same as what would have occurred without our observation. The Hawthorne Effect is best avoided by a study design in which both the treatment and the control groups are equally aware of their participation in a study.

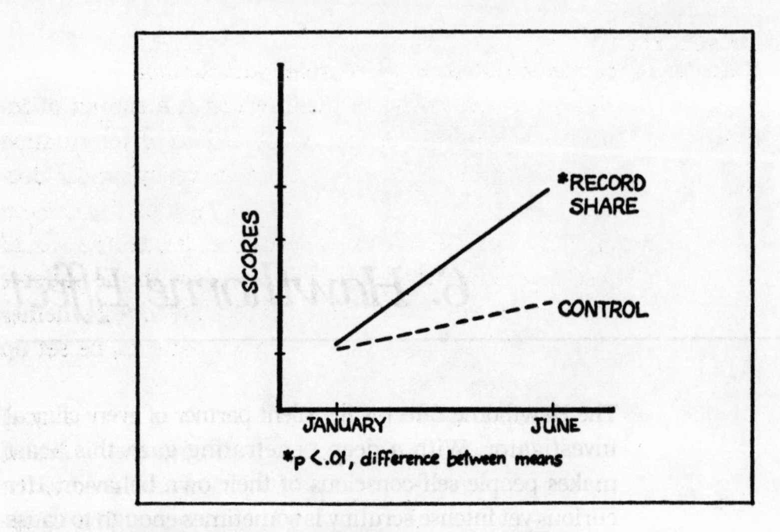

Figure 2. Patient satisfaction scores, study 1.

CASE STUDY
Access to the Medical Record and Patient Satisfaction

Patient access to the medical record is a subject of increasing debate since the 1973 Freedom of Information Act removed the aura of secrecy from many similar documents. In early 1980, Dr. Wa'Na Peek of the Oregon People's Center for Herbal Medicine decided he would like to routinely share medical records with the patients in his clinic. Recognizing the opportunity to test whether record sharing was beneficial to his patients, he set up the following study.

One hundred consecutive patients were given a brief questionnaire regarding satisfaction with their medical care. These patients were then randomly assigned to the "treatment" group or to the "control" group. The 50 patients in the treatment group were given ten minutes in the examination room to read their own medical record and were then invited to ask questions about its contents. The other 50 patients went through the usual office routine without seeing their records. At the end of six months both groups were again administered the satisfaction questionnaire.

As shown in Figure 2 the two groups had comparable satisfaction scores at the start of the study. Six months later the record-sharing group had a significant increase in their scores, indicating a positive influence of access to the medical record.

Dr. Peek found the results of his study persuasive and presented these data at a staff meeting at the center. On the basis of his data he began to make plans to extend record sharing to all his patients, and his results were published as a lead article in the *Yin/Yang Journal of Wellness.*

Comment

Dr. Wa'Na Peek's data show an increase in patient satisfaction. Is that change specifically due to record sharing or is it because the patients in the treatment group were given more attention in the office? When this question was raised at the staff meeting, Dr. Peek decided to conduct a second study.

Another 100 patients were given the satisfaction questionnaire. As in the first study, half were given their medical record and the opportunity to ask questions. This time, however, the control group was also given the chance to ask questions about their health concerns and their medical care. Specific discussion of the medical record itself was avoided.

After six months the satisfaction questionnaire was readministered to all 100 patients. Much to Dr. Peek's surprise the results were different this time.

Both groups demonstrated a significant improvement in satisfaction rating at the end of six months (Fig. 3). Dr. Peek astutely noted that the results were caused by the Hawthorne Effect; simply showing interest in what the patient thought, whether it concerned his medical record or his medical care in general, was enough to improve satisfaction. Had the second study not been done, Dr. Peek might have given credit to record sharing for the improvement, when in fact the credit belonged to him, for his added show of concern for his patients.

The Hawthorne Effect was first spotted outside a Western Electric plant near Chicago in the early 1930's [1]. Efforts by the company officials to improve productivity led to very confusing results since just about any change in working conditions, even neutral changes, increased productivity. Eventually what came to be called the Hawthorne Effect was recognized as the culprit. Showing an interest in the employees was enough to change their working behavior and increase production.

In any study of behavior or attitude, care must be taken to avoid the very human proclivity to be affected by observation. The dialogue between researcher and patient, doctor and patient, or even researcher and doctor, is where the Hawthorne Effect works her changes. For ex-

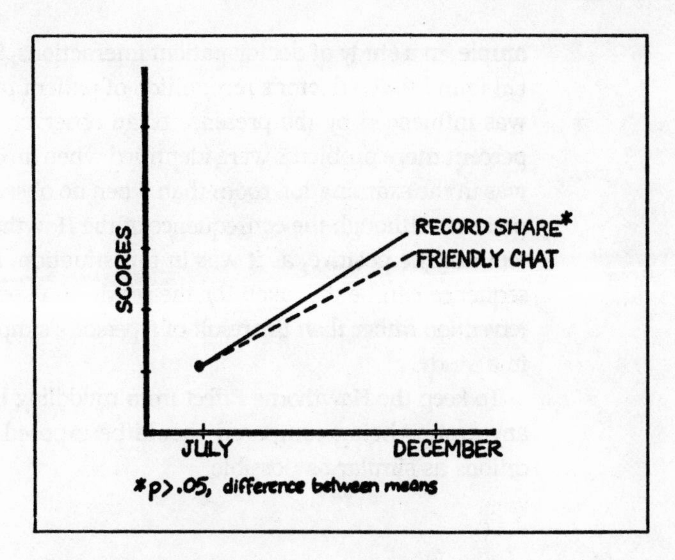

Figure 3. Patient satisfaction scores, study 2.

ample, in a study of doctor-patient interactions, Starfield [2] found that a doctor's recognition of patient problems was influenced by the presence of an observer. Twenty percent more problems were identified when an observer was in the examination room than when no observer was present. Although the consequence of the Hawthorne Effect may be positive, as it was in this situation, the consequence can be mistaken for the result of a specific intervention rather than the result of a person's simply being in a study.

To keep the Hawthorne Effect from muddling the data, any groups being compared should be exposed to conditions as similar as possible.

EXAMPLES

Bertera, E. M., and Bertera, R. L. The cost effectiveness of telephone vs. clinic counseling for hypertensive patients: A pilot study. *Am. J. Public Health* 71:626, 1981.

This study evaluates the effect of telephone- and clinic-based counseling on blood pressure control in hypertensive patients. Significant improvement in blood pressure control was found in patients who received telephone or clinic counseling when compared to a large clinic control group. The authors conclude that this change resulted from the counseling and its content. However, the time spent with each patient may have resulted in better blood pressure control regardless of what was discussed during that time. Any contact with a representative of the clinic may have led to the same effect.

Earp, J. A., Ory, M., and Strogats, D. S. The effects of family involvement and practitioner home visits on the control of hypertension. *Am. J. Public Health* 72:1146, 1982.

Hypertensive patients who received care from home-visiting health practitioners or from family members were compared to patients who received routine clinic care. Patients were placed in one of three randomly selected groups. At one year all three groups were similar in blood pressure control; at two years there was slightly improved control in the two study groups. Although a great deal of effort was expended in patient education, the results may be explained in part by the Hawthorne Effect.

Martin, A. R., Wolf, M. A., Thibadleau, L. A., et al. A trial of two strategies to modify the test-ordering behavior of medical residents. *N. Engl. J. Med.* 303:1330, 1980.

Three teams of medical residents were told of an ongoing study to alter test-ordering. Two groups received different incentives to modify the number of tests ordered; a third group served as a control. The two study groups had a significant decline in test ordering when compared to the control group, which showed little change. Six months after the conclusion of the study the two study groups continued to order fewer tests. These results indicate that the changes were an effect of the intervention, rather than a consequence of the Hawthorne Effect, since change due to the Hawthorne Effect would tend to disappear soon after the trial ended.

McDonald, C. J., Wilson, G. A., and McCabe, G. P. Physician response to computer reminders. *J.A.M.A.* 244:1579, 1980.

A computerized record system used in a clinic setting reminded physicians about findings (e.g., abnormal laboratory values) that might need attention. Three phases—a control period and two interventions—were studied in all of the six possible temporal orders to elicit the "educational" effect of the reminders. By exposing the subjects to all interventions at some point in the study the Hawthorne Effect was avoided, and the differences in results could be properly attributed to the computer reminder system.

Rhyne, R. and Gelbach, S. H. Effects of educational feedback strategy on physician utilization of thyroid function panels. *J. Fam. Pract.* 8:1003, 1979.

An educational program to influence ordering of thyroid function panels was initially quite effective, reducing the rate these tests were ordered by 35 percent. Within several months, however, the number of thyroid tests ordered had returned to previous levels. The authors attributed the initial change to the Hawthorne Effect rather than to information learned in the program.

REFERENCES

1. Sonnenfield, J. Hawthorne: Illuminations and illusions. *Harvard Business Review* 58:51, 1982.
2. Starfield, B., Steinwachs, D., Morris, J., et al. Presence of observers at patient-practitioner interactions: Impact on coordination of care and methodologic implications. *Am. J. Public Health* 69:1021, 1979.

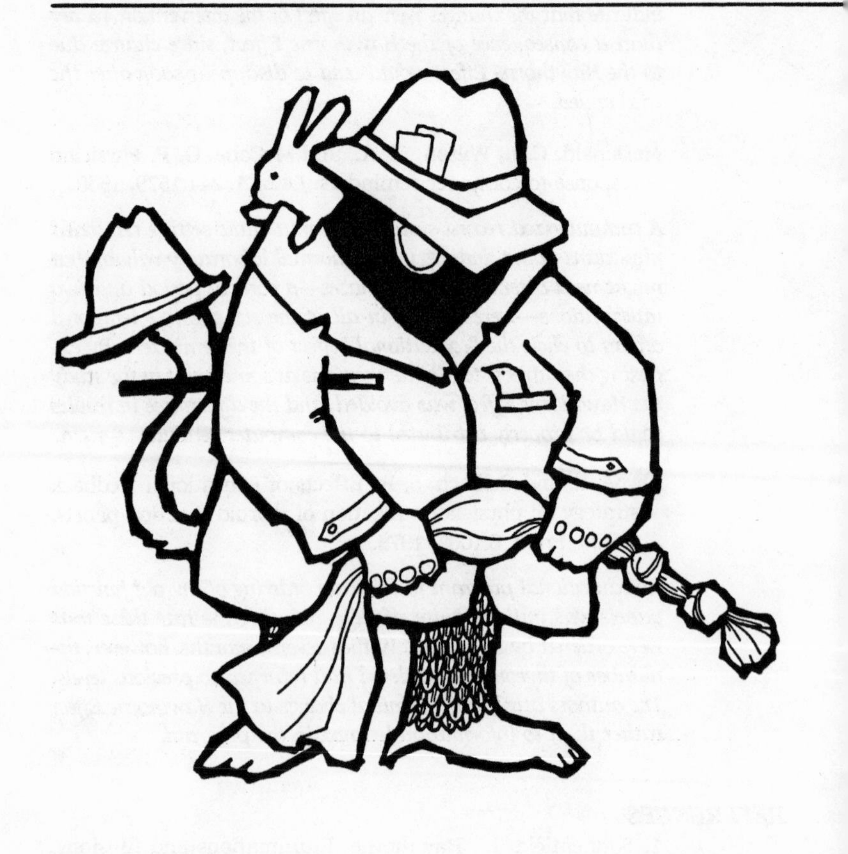

7. Diagnostic Accuracy Bias

Diagnostic Accuracy Bias is the con man of the biomedical bestiary. This greasy little fellow preys on physicians' innate predisposition to see what they expect to see (a predisposition on which physicians have no monopoly). His sleight of hand capitalizes on our tendency to attribute changes in the rate of a disease to alterations in its cause or therapy. He cleverly hides from us the possibility that a change in a disease rate may be only an apparition, an artifact of changes in the way we make or think about a diagnosis. Keep an eye on your hat when reading a paper describing recent changes in the incidence of a disease; Diagnostic Accuracy Bias may well be in the vicinity.

DEFINITION

Diagnostic accuracy bias refers to the tendency to attribute changes in the incidence of a disease to changes in therapeutic efficacy or to changes in exposure to factors that cause the disease. Often, changes in the incidence of a disease are only apparent; the actual change is in the means by which the disease is identified.

CASE STUDY
Diverticulitis in Strawberry Fields

At the 1981 meeting of the North American Society for Integrative Healing, Dr. Arnold Kadette presented results

of a study examining secular trends in the incidence of diverticulitis is an isolated northern California community. Strawberry Fields, a multi-generational community of 20,000 people, was incorporated in 1960 with the intent of offering, in the words of its charter, "a pastoral lifestyle for the Aquarian era." Dr. J. M. Space, a retired allergist, was hired by the community when it opened and, over a period of two decades, kept detailed records of his clinical observations on the incidences of various diseases in Strawberry Fields.

Dr. Kadette's analysis of these records revealed a fascinating observation. The yearly incidence of diverticulitis was nearly constant until 1972, when there was a marked decline in the appearance of new cases (Fig. 4).

Intrigued by this observation, Dr. Kadette compared the therapeutic efficacy of treatment of new cases of diverticulitis diagnosed in 1965 with those diagnosed in 1975. As shown in Table 8, the resolution of symptoms and the likelihood of recurrence was markedly better in the 1975 group of patients than in the 1965 group. Since no alterations had been made in Dr. Space's therapeutic approach to diverticulitis, Dr. Kadette inferred that a radical change had occurred in the population's exposure to some important etiologic or protective factor.

Reviewing the notes of community meetings, Dr. Space recalled that in 1971 the Community Wellness Coalition had begun a massive campaign to educate the community regarding "the importance of dietary fiber." So successful was this project that the per capita consumption of granola tripled by January of 1972. Dr. Kadette hypothesized that the marked increase in the community's intake of granola was responsible for the decline in diverticulitis attacks and the improvement in therapeutic response among diverticulitis patients.

Comments

As clinicians interested in the causes and treatment of disease, we have an almost reflexive tendency to view

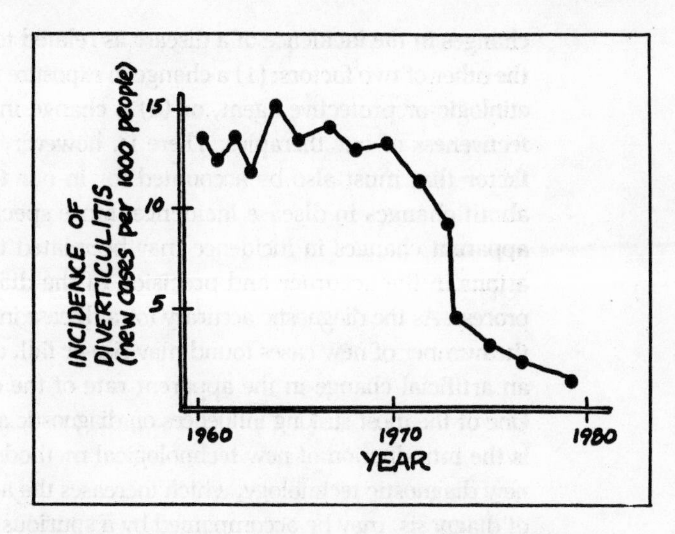

Figure 4. Incidence of diverticulitis in Strawberry Fields, 1960–1980.

Table 8. Symptom resolution and recurrence in diverticulitis patients

Year	Number of cases	Mean number of days to resolution of symptoms	Recurrence of symptoms within 6 months (%)
1965	240	31	10
1975	100	6	1

changes in the incidence of a disease as related to one or the other of two factors: (1) a change in exposure to some etiologic or protective agent, or (2) a change in the effectiveness of our therapies. There is, however, a third factor that must also be accounted for in our thinking about changes in disease incidence. More specifically, apparent changes in incidence may be related to alterations in the accuracy and precision of the diagnostic process. As the diagnostic accuracy for a disease improves, the number of new cases found may rise or fall, creating an artificial change in the apparent rate of the disease. One of the most striking influences on diagnostic accuracy is the introduction of new technological methods. Thus, new diagnostic technology, which increases the accuracy of diagnosis, may be accompanied by a spurious change in the incidence of a disease.

The major omission in the analysis of the Strawberry Fields data was the failure to assess changes in the diagnostic process that might have accounted for the decline in diverticulitis. Further perusal of the Strawberry Fields community records revealed that in 1971 a fiberoptic colonoscope was donated to Dr. Space by the New Age Kiwanis Club. Thereafter, patients presenting with colicky abdominal pain and a change in bowel habits enjoyed the benefits of colonoscopy as part of their diagnostic workup. In previous years, the diagnosis of diverticulitis was made, and appropriate therapeutic regimen prescribed, on clinical grounds alone.

The fall in diagnoses of diverticulitis after 1972 was accompanied by a concurrent increase in diagnoses of other colonic diseases (Fig. 5). The change in the incidence of diverticulitis was related principally to the introduction of a new diagnostic instrument that permitted the detection of a number of heretofore occult conditions, such as polyps, cancer, and irritable colon.

What about the documented change in therapeutic response for patients with a diagnosis of diverticulitis? Remember that in 1965 a number of patients labelled with the diagnosis of "diverticulitis" were probably really suf-

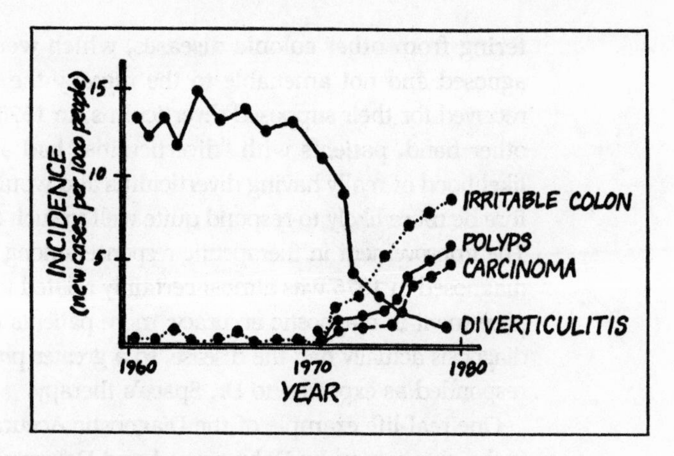

Figure 5. Incidence of diverticulitis, irritable colon, polyps, and carcinoma in Strawberry Fields, 1960–1980.

fering from other colonic diseases, which were undiagnosed and not amenable to the therapy the patients received for their supposed diverticulitis. In 1975, on the other hand, patients with "diverticulitis" had a greater likelihood of really having diverticulitis and would therefore be more likely to respond quite well to such therapy. The improvement in therapeutic response among patients diagnosed in 1975 was almost certainly related to an improvement in diagnostic accuracy: more patients with the diagnosis actually had the disease, so a greater proportion responded as expected to Dr. Space's therapy.

One real-life example of the Diagnostic Accuracy Bias is the observation by Dohrenwend and Dohrenwend [1] that the reported prevalence of psychiatric disorders changed markedly from the years prior to World War II (3.6%) to the years immediately following the war (20%). Their analysis indicates that the diffference in results is attributable, at least in part, to the effects of nomenclature changes on the rates of mental disorders counted in communities.

Two more examples are (1) the marked increase in the discernment of dysmorphological features in Native American children following the initial description of fetal alcohol syndrome, and (2) the striking increase in the antemortem identification of atherosclerotic heart disease in the late 1920s, following the introduction of the electrocardiogram as a diagnostic tool.

Technological advances that increase the accuracy of diagnosis or shifts in conventions regarding the naming of diseases can both be accompanied by marked changes in the rate of a disease and its apparent response to therapy. Keep this in mind, lest you become another of the innocent victims deceived by Diagnostic Accuracy Bias.

SUGGESTED READING

Feinstein, A. R. Clinical epidemiology: II. The identification rates of disease. *Ann. Intern. Med.* 69:1037, 1968.

This is a definitive review of factors influencing the identification of disease, including nomenclature, diagnostic criteria, and the introduction of new technology. Feinstein provides a good historic example of the apparent changes in disease rates that can accompany the dissemination of a new diagnostic technique. Around 1919, a decline began in the United States in deaths attributed to bronchitis and pneumonia, while at the same time a striking increase occurred in deaths related to cancer of the lung. The apparent changes in the rates of disease were probably a result of improvements in roentgenography between 1920 and 1940 and the increasing use of diagnostic chest x-rays.

Feinstein, A. R. The Rancid Sample, the Tilted Target, and the Medical Pallbearer. In A. R. Feinstein, *Clinical Biostatistics.* St. Louis: Mosby, 1977.

This is a more detailed discussion of the above topic.

REFERENCE

1. Dohrenwend, B. P., and Dohrenwend, B. S. Perspectives on the past and future of psychiatric epidemiology. *Am. J. Public Health* 72:1271, 1982.

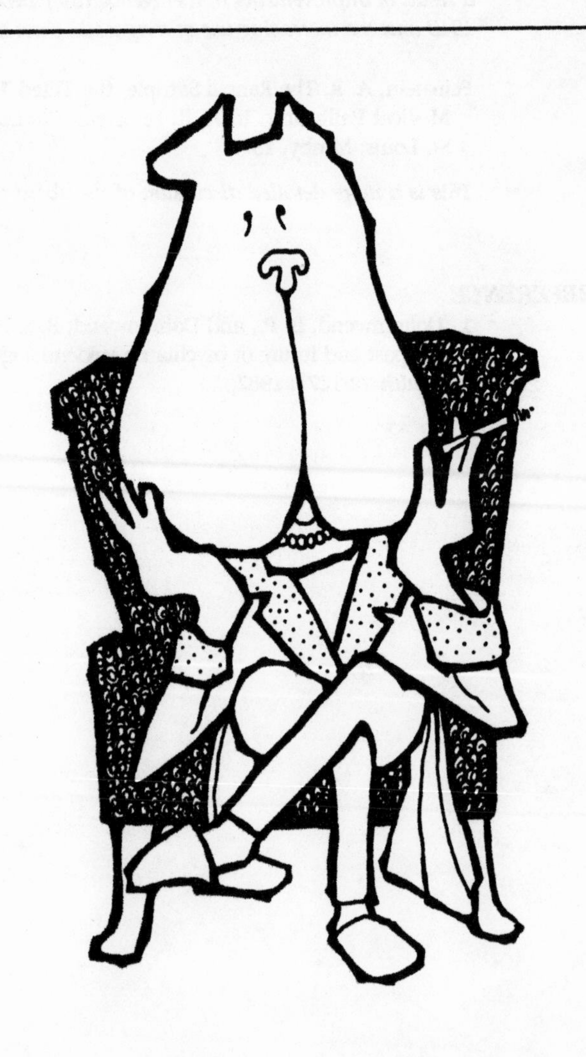

8. Regression Meany

The Regression Meany is a consummate bore. He is the sort of fellow who, armed with dull wit and narcoleptic personality, can turn the most exciting, outlandish tale into a colorless report. Fifteen well-spent minutes with this tedious creature are guaranteed to induce somnolence in all but the hardiest listeners. He fouls the medical literature by creating a predisposition for interesting or abnormal findings to go away. Specifically, he causes subjects who are at the extremes of a biological spectrum to drift toward normal, more boring, values on later measurements. This predisposition—known as regression to the mean—enables the Regression Meany to trick us into concluding that meaningful change has occurred. All we may have witnessed, however, is the tendency for exciting extremes to be reduced to bland mediocrities by the soporific influence of this boring little beast.

DEFINITION

Regression to the mean is the tendency for individuals with very high or very low scores on one measurement of a variable to have scores closer to the center of the distribution when measured a second time.

CASE STUDY
Incentives and Nurse Practitioners

Dr. Stanley Hubris of the Out West Institute for Health Services Research studied one hundred family nurse practitioners (FNPs) practicing in the state of Nevada. During a two-month period, visits were made to nurses at their clinical sites in order to assess their performance of various medical tasks and skills, including history taking, physical examination, clinical judgment, and use of the medical record. In addition, a written test of general medical knowledge was given to each FNP on the day of the site visit. All scores were then combined into a cumulative index of performance. The 15 FNPs receiving the highest scores were given $500 and an engraved plaque for their offices, and their names were published in the *FNP Quarterly*.

The next year, the same battery of tests was administered to the same 100 FNPs. To Dr. Hubris's surprise, the average score of the rewarded FNPs dropped five percent, while the average score for all 100 improved by 10 percent (Fig. 6)!

Hubris then began a second study using the same tests and procedures as in the first, but this time he employed a system of *negative* incentives for those with poor scores. The fifteen FNPs with the lowest scores on the second set of tests were denied both their usual free subscription to *FNP Quarterly* and their annual pay raise. When retested the following year, the 15 punished FNPs average score increased by 20 percent, while the score for the entire 100 increased by only 5 percent (Fig. 7).

Dr. Hubris concluded, in his well-known paper, "Pride and Punishment of FNPs," that nurse practitioners respond best to a negative incentive plan. He speculated that this may be related to unresolved guilt engendered by their assumption of a role previously allowed only to the M.D.

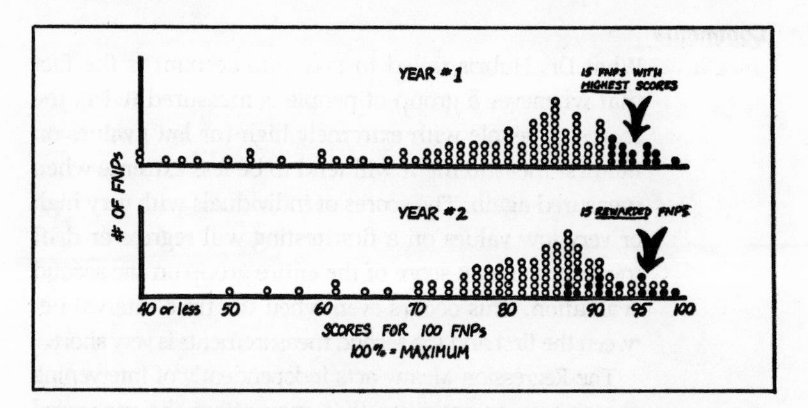

Figure 6. Family nurse practitioner test scores, years 1 and 2.

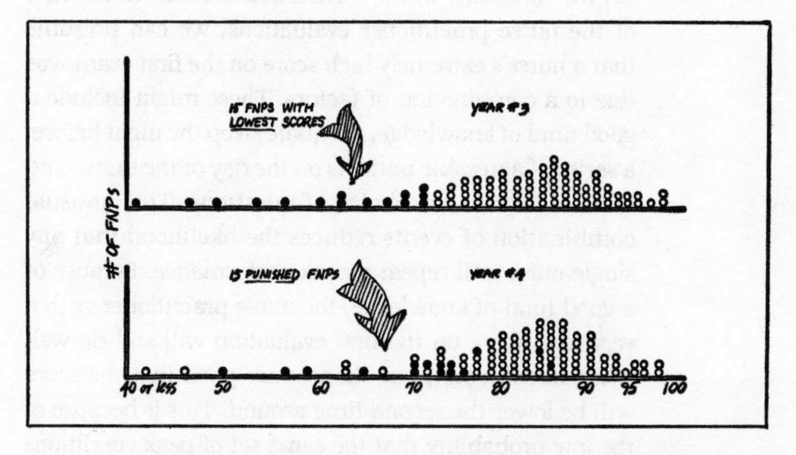

Figure 7. Family nurse practitioner test scores, years 3 and 4.

Comments

What Dr. Hubris failed to take into account is the fact that whenever a group of people is measured twice, the scores of people with extremely high (or low) values on the first measurement will tend to be less extreme when measured again. The scores of individuals with very high or very low values on a first testing will regress or drift toward the mean score of the entire group on the second evaluation. This occurs even when the time interval between the first and the second measurements is very short.

The Regression Meany acts independently of intervening experiences or activities that may affect the measured characteristic. Instead, regression is caused by the combined effects of two sources of variability: (1) the variability inherent in the characteristic being measured, and (2) the variability in the measurement itself. In the case of the nurse practitioner evaluations, we can presume that a nurse's extremely high score on the first exam was due to a combination of factors. These might include a good fund of knowledge, adequate sleep the night before, a series of agreeable patients on the day of the exam, and a bit of luck in the choice of questions. This unusual combination of events reduces the likelihood that any single nurse will repeat a peak performance. Because of a good fund of knowledge, the nurse practitioner with a very high score on the first evaluation will still do well when tested again, but chances are good that the score will be lower the second time around. This is because of the low probability that the same set of peak conditions will exist again the second time.

There are many studies in the medical literature in which the Regression Meany may play an important role. Common to each is the potential for wrongly inferring that an observed change is due to some medically important cause, like aging, or the natural course of the disease, or the effect of a therapeutic agent. For example, an uncontrolled test of a new drug given to hypertensive patients may show a significant decline in blood pressure that is attributable only to the inherent tendency for later measurements to be lower than the earlier measurements by which the patients were initially diagnosed. Unless a control group is also measured, we would be unable to distinguish drug effects from regression to the mean.

A real example of the regression effect may have occurred in a study by Paradise and associates published in 1978 [1]. Sixty-five children with presenting histories of frequent, recurrent, throat infections were followed prospectively for the development of subsequent episodes. During the first year of close observation, only 11 children (17%) had throat infections with the same frequency and clinical features as described in their histories. Of the remaining 54 children, 80 percent experienced a negligible number of infections. The authors attributed the discrepancy between the historical data and the follow-up observations to a number of possible explanations, including change in the incidence of infection with increasing age and parental exaggeration of the illness history. It is also possible, however, that regression to the mean could have accounted for some of the change in illness frequency.

Watch your step around studies that single out an extreme group for observation! You may be wrongly convinced that real change has occurred, when in fact the Regression Meany has lured those exciting extremes into mediocre submission.

EXAMPLES

Ederer, F. Serum cholesterol changes: Effects of diet and regression toward the mean. *J. Chronic Dis.* 25:277, 1972.

This is a theoretical discussion of regression to the mean in studies of dietary influences on serum cholesterol. The author presents a mathematical method for separating dietary and regression effects.

Fixler, S. E., Laird, W. P., Fitzgerald, V., et al. Hypertension screening in the schools: Results of the Dallas study. *Pediatrics* 63:32, 1979.

This is another good example of the Regression Meany. Of 947 students with an elevated reading on a first screening measurement, only 167 had subsequent readings suggestive of persistent hypertension.

Glasunov, I. S., Dowd, J. E., Jaksić, Z., et al. Repetitive health examinations as an intervention measure. *Bull. WHO* 49:423, 1973.

Levels of systolic blood pressure, cholesterol, and glucose showed a substantial decrease over a period of two years in both a medication-treated group and a control group. The authors discuss the possibility that at least some of the improvement could be accounted for by regression to the mean.

Huck, S. W., and Sandler, H. M. *Rival Hypotheses: Alternative Interpretations of Data Based Conclusions.* New York: Harper & Row, 1979. Pp. 94, 196–197.

These authors discuss the criticism of early studies that purported to show that Project Head Start had little or no effect on children's educational achievement. They point out, however, that in at least one study Head Start children were matched with children in other preschools on the basis of IQ. Because it would have been more difficult to find matches for the most disadvantaged children, it is likely that children at the upper end of the IQ distribution in Head Start classes were matched with children at the lower end in regular preschools. "Thus," as Huck and Sandler wrote, "both samples being compared were extreme relative to their respective populations. Any time the samples are chosen as a consequence of being extreme, we can expect to find the statistical artifact of regression toward the mean."

Laskarzewski, P., Morrison, J. A., deGroot, I., et al. Lipid and lipoprotein tracking in 108 children over a four-year period. *Pediatrics* 64:584, 1979.

In this paper, the authors have used statistical methods to separate regression effects from actual changes in a measured biological parameter.

SUGGESTED READING

Davis, C. E. The effect of regression to the mean in epidemiologic and clinical studies. *Am. J. Epidemiol.* 104:493, 1976.

Davis's review article is perhaps the best overall discussion of the regression phenomenon and the statistical methods available for controlling for its effect.

Furby, L. Interpreting regression toward the mean in developmental research. *Dev. Psychol.* 8:172, 1973.

This is an analysis of the regression phenomenon in the study of developmental change.

Nesselroade, J. R., Stigler, S. M., and Baltes, P. B. Regression toward the mean and the study of change. *Psychol. Bull.* 88:622, 1980.

Another good review article. Nesselroade argues that regression to the mean is not *a ubiquitous phenomenon and that its consideration should depend on the underlying model of the process being studied.*

REFERENCE

1. Paradise, J. L., Bluestone, C. D., Bachman, R. Z., et al. History of recurrent sore throat as an indication for tonsillectomy. *N. Engl. J. Med.* 298:409, 1978.

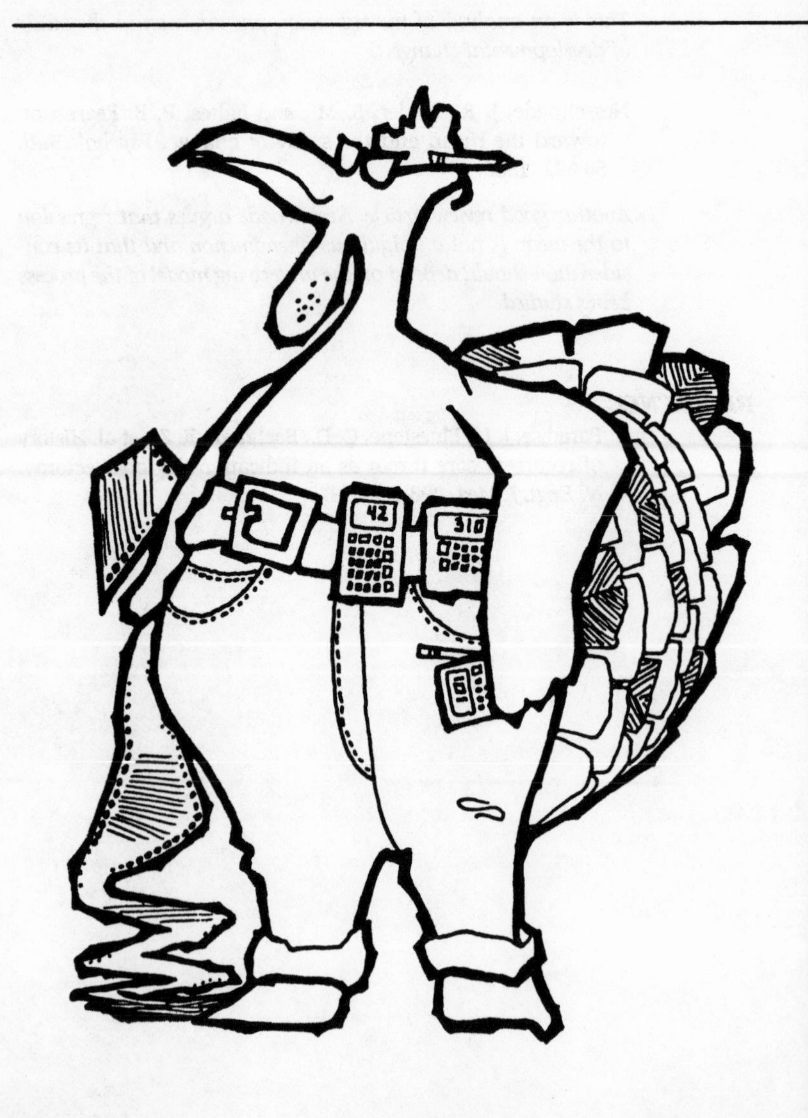

9. *Significance Turkey*

Peering at you from behind greasy lenses, the beady-eyed Significance Turkey is extremely impressed with the numbers he has generated. Armed with several varieties of pocket calculators strapped to his belt and mountains of computer printouts, he stands before you hawking *p*-values. Vacant of mind and totally out of touch with the living world, he is, in short, a biostatistical bozo. Be careful, however, with this pubescent prodigy: his methods are mathematical and smack of the Science in which we are such true and indiscriminate believers. His beloved numbers can blind you.

DEFINITION

Tests of *statistical significance* assess the possibility that an apparent association between one variable (e.g., a disease) and another (e.g., a possible etiologic agent) is really due only to the effect of chance. Judgments of *clinical importance*, on the other hand, evaluate the magnitude of the association and ask the question: Even if the association is statistically significant, is it large enough to make any real difference to patients or their physicians? A statistically significant association is not necessarily a clinically important association.

Table 9. Incidence of prostatitis in 10,000 New Foundland businessmen by exposure to Cornish game hens over 30-year period

Group	Prostatitis cases	Non-cases
Hen eaters	48	9,952
Hen avoiders	30*	9,970

*$\chi^2 = 4.2, p < .05$

CASE STUDIES

Cornish Game Hens and Prostatitis

In a recent paper appearing in the prestigious *New FoundlandJournal of Medicine*, Dr. Ralph Nadir reported an increased risk of prostatitis among regular consumers of Cornish game hens. Beginning with case reports of severe prostatitis among chicken farmers and the known appetite of game hens for all manner of industrial wastes, Dr. Nadir speculated that the flesh of these birds might have inflammatory properties. In 1950, two cohorts of New Foundland businessmen were enrolled in a 30-year follow-up study. One cohort was selected on the basis of a dietary history of three to five game hens eaten weekly, while the other cohort was selected on the basis of the subjects' strong aversion to eating birds. Dr. Nadir's detailed review of other dietary factors, personal habits, industrial exposures, and social class showed that the two cohorts were almost identical with respect to other known risk factors for the development of prostatitis. Table 9 summarizes the results of the 30-year surveillance.

Dr. Nadir's data indicate a statistically significant increase in the risk of prostatitis among consumers of Cornish game hens. As a result, the World Health Organization has added game hens to its growing list of dietary hazards, and the American Urological Society has publicly advocated the deportation of all hens currently residing within the United States and its territories.

Computers and IQ Scores

Increasingly, national attention has focused on the use of computer technology in the educational process. Dr. Kyle Square of the Bronx Cybernetic Association (BCA) has completed a randomized controlled trial of an intensive, computer-based curriculum for elementary school children. Dr. Square's study leaves no doubt as to the efficacy of this instructional package in raising levels of academic performance.

Table 10. Pre- and post-intervention IQ scores among Bronx school children

Study Group	Mean scores on Stanford-Binet Wide Range Achievement Test (range)		
	Enrollment	May	September
Experimental (computer curriculum)	4,000	105.0(83–137)	107.8(83–141)
Control	4,000	105.1(82–142)	105.5*(85–139)

*By t-test for difference between means, $p < .001$

Eight thousand Bronx school children were randomly assigned to one of two summer camps. At the experimental camp, children spent three months in an intensive, 10-hour-per-day, computer course designed to increase general knowledge. At the control camp, children engaged in the usual, generally unproductive, camp activities such as swimming, hiking, sailing, and goofing-off. Summer programs at both camps were well-received, with only minor insurrections and sporadic runaways at the experimental site. (Square noted that "school-age children are known for their distrust of new and innovative programs.") Analysis of data confirmed that the experimental and control group populations were identical at the time of enrollment with respect to age, sex, and race distributions, baseline IQs, and past school performance.

Table 10 shows the results of pre- and post-summer testing for children at both camps. Strikingly apparent is the statistically significant increase in IQ scores among experimental group children. Dr. Square and the BCA concluded that computer camps for children are highly effective approaches to maximizing the academic achievements of school children.

Comments

The statistical significance of a difference between outcome scores for two groups of subjects is determined by a combination of the size of the difference, the size of the groups, and the variability in their scores. As a consequence, extremely small study populations can prove little, while very large populations can prove many things. Thus, even when the difference in outcomes is extraordinarily small, it may still be "significant" if the groups studied are extraordinarily large.

Such was the case in the fabled projects of Drs. Nadir and Square. In Dr. Nadir's study, eating Cornish game hens raised the likelihood of developing prostatitis by 18 chances in 10,000—a negligible increase in risk, but significant by virtue of Dr. Nadir's cast of thousands. Similarly, Dr. Square raised IQs by over two points in his experimental group of children, proving that even the most clinically *in*significant difference can emerge as statistically significant if the study is big enough.

Listen for the pedantic gobbling of the Significance Turkey. After he has shown you his gaggle of numbers, proving beyond anyone's reasonable doubt the statistical significance of his findings, remember that *your* task is to assess the clinical importance of his study. No *p*-value, no matter how small, ever proved that a research result was *important.*

EXAMPLES

Qvarnberg, Y. Acute otitis media: A prospective clinical study of myringotomy and antimicrobial treatment. *Acta Otolaryngol.* [Suppl.] 375, 1981.

Almost 250 children with acute otitis media were randomized into a controlled trial of three different interventions: (1) penicillin alone, (2) amoxicillin alone, and (3) penicillin plus myringotomy. At the end of three months, 15 percent of those children treated with antibiotics alone still had abnormal findings on an ear examination, compared with 4 percent of those in whom a myringotomy was also done. Although this difference in long-term outcome was statistically *significant, one wonders whether the 11 percent decrease in persistent abnormalities is sufficient to clinically justify the pain and difficulty of myringotomy. Even in the short-term, where a nearly* 25 percent *difference in resolution was found, the* clinical *importance of the difference remains open to question.*

Tuthill, R. W., and Calabrese, E. J. Elevated sodium levels in the public drinking water as a contributor to elevated blood pressure levels in the community. *Arch. Environ. Health* 34:197, 1974.

Blood pressure measurements among 600 high school sophomores in two similar communities were compared. The primary difference between the two communities was in the level of sodium contained in drinking water. Students from the high-sodium community showed a statistically significant elevation in mean blood pressure: 2.7 mmHg for boys and 5.1 mmHg for girls. While such differences in blood pressure levels may be important from a public health standpoint, it is unlikely that the differences would be clinically *important for the individual child.*

SUGGESTED READING

Feinstein, A. R. *Clinical Biostatistics.* St. Louis: Mosby, 1977. Chap. 18.

This book contains a good review of the distinction between statistical significance and clinical or therapeutic importance.

Freiman, J. A. The importance of beta, the type II error and sample size in the design and interpretation of the randomized control trial. *N. Engl. J. Med.* 299:828, 1978.

This paper provides a very good discussion of type II errors in randomized control trials, that is, studies in which a true difference between groups is not discovered because of an inadequate population size (see also Chapter 10, Nerd of Nonsignificance).

Murphy, E. A. *The Logic of Medicine.* Baltimore: Johns Hopkins University Press, 1976.

Murphy's work is mandatory reading for physicians and others interested in the structure and logic of medical thinking.

Sackett, D. L. How to read clinical journals: V. To distinguish useful from useless or even harmful therapy. *Can. Med. Assoc. J.* 124:1156, 1981.

This excellent paper contains a discussion of the difference between statistical significance and clinical importance and the determinants of each.

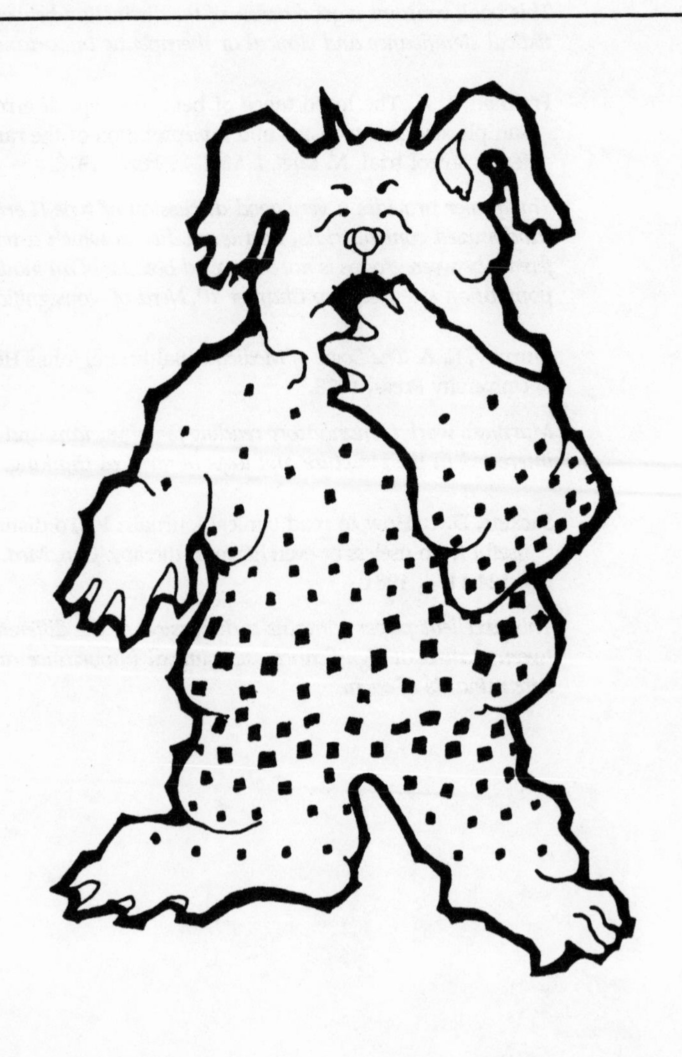

10. Nerd of Nonsignificance

The Nerd of Nonsignificance is the nemesis of studies too small to test their hypotheses. The Nerd's view of the world is limp, dreary, and spiritless. He expects that nothing interesting can ever happen to him, and nothing ever does. How could this ineffectual soul be a menace? He manages to mislead us by shrugging off every finding that is not statistically significant. He assumes that if a result isn't statistically significant, it must be meaningless. In doing so, he fails to realize that his own lack of power could be at fault.

DEFINITION

The power of a study to detect a real finding is determined by the size of the finding and by the size of the study sample. Where the sample size is very large, even a very small finding can be statistically significant. Conversely, when the sample size is relatively small, a large finding may be statistically nonsignificant, even when it is clinically or therapeutically important. To conclude on the basis of a statistical test that there is no meaningful finding in such a case may be to overlook a useful clue concerning a real effect.

CASE STUDY
Cadaver's Revenge

Toxicologists have recently noted that rats exposed to formaldehyde fumes have a high risk of developing cancers of the nasopharynx. Since formaldehyde is a common industrial chemical, its potential as a human carcinogen has become a matter of immediate concern. Dr. Mortimer Titian found himself in an ideal position to test the hypothesis. Only last year, he had completed a study of heart disease among 305 undertakers. Dr. Titian had collected data on all illnesses among his undertaker sample, but had never specifically analyzed cancer. Undertakers are frequently exposed to formaldehyde in the form of embalming fluid. Thus, they form an ideal group of persons on which to test the cancer hypothesis.

Fully recognizing this important opportunity, Dr. Titian reviewed his original data and compared the rates of nasopharyngeal cancer among the undertakers to his control group (Table 11). With a *p*-value of .09, there was no significant difference in risk between the two groups. Dr. Titian was disappointed, but dutifully wrote up a report that appeared in the *Midwest Journal of Mortuary Sciences*.

Two years later, a large study of medical pathologists was published. The findings are shown in Table 12. These authors concluded that pathologists were three times as likely to develop nasopharyngeal cancer as unexposed persons, and that formaldehyde was a human carcinogen.

In some confusion, Dr. Titian dug out his old computer printouts. Belatedly, he realized that the undertakers' risk was also elevated threefold over his controls. However, because his study was only a third the size of the pathologist study, the difference between the cases and the controls was not statistically significant. His attention to the *p*-value had caused him to ignore a strongly suggestive finding in a study too small to provide a statistically significant result.

Table 11. Risk of nasopharyngeal cancer among undertakers

Study group	Incidence of nasopharyngeal cancer
Undertakers	9/305 (3%)
Control	3/306 (1%)

$p = .09$

Table 12. Risk of nasopharyngeal cancer among medical pathologists

Study group	Incidence of nasopharyngeal cancer
Pathologists	32/1,023 (3%)
Control	13/1,101 (1%)

$p < .01$

Comment

Although the formaldehyde study is fictitious, the problem is not uncommon. Data from samples that are too small to detect a significant difference must be interpreted cautiously. "Not statistically significant" does not mean "not important"; it merely means the finding could well be due to chance.

For several years the effect of mothers' smoking on perinatal mortality was in dispute, partly because the studies conducted had been too small to consistently show a statistically significant result. In the case of perinatal deaths, which are uncommon, even a large study could be relatively too small to demonstrate the modest increase in risk that really exists. In 1971, a study was published that included data from 3,290 black infants. Among this group, infants of mothers who smoked had 26 percent higher mortality than infants of nonsmokers. However, this difference was not statistically significant, and the author concluded that "no increase in neonatal mortality was noted" [1]. Later papers with much larger study populations reported statistically significant increases of 28 percent [2] and 20 to 35 percent mortality [3] associated with mothers' smoking. Thus, the 26 percent increase observed in the first paper was probably not due to chance, even if it was not significant.

The ability of a study to detect a difference that really exists is known as its power. A study's power depends on several factors, especially sample size and the size of the difference that is being measured. The power of a study can be estimated even before it is carried out, using readily available mathematical formulas [4]. Before a study is begun, the careful researcher will do those power calculations to make sure there is a reasonable chance of statistically detecting the hypothesized difference, assuming it exists. In any analysis, the possibility of a false-negative statistical finding must always be considered. The Nerd of Nonsignificance is quick to brush off a finding that may later prove to have been important.

SUGGESTED READING

Mainland, D. The significance of "non-significance." *Clin. Pharmacol. Ther.* 4:580, 1963.

This is a straightforward discussion of statistical test interpretation, written by a statistician for non-statisticians.

REFERENCES

1. Yerushalmy, J. The relationship of parents' cigarette smoking to the outcome of pregnancy. Implications as to the problem of inferring causation from observed associations: *Am. J. Epidemiol.* 93:443, 1971.
2. Butler, N. R., Goldstein, H., and Ross, E. M. Cigarette smoking in pregnancy: Its influence on birthweight and perinatal mortality. *Br. Med. J.* 2:127, 1972.
3. Meyer, M. B., Jonas, B. S., and Tonascia, J. A. Perinatal events associated with maternal smoking during pregnancy. *Am. J. Epidemiol.* 103:464, 1976.
4. Schlesselman, J. J. Sample size requirements in cohort and case-control studies of disease, *Am. J. Epidemiol.* 99:381, 1974.

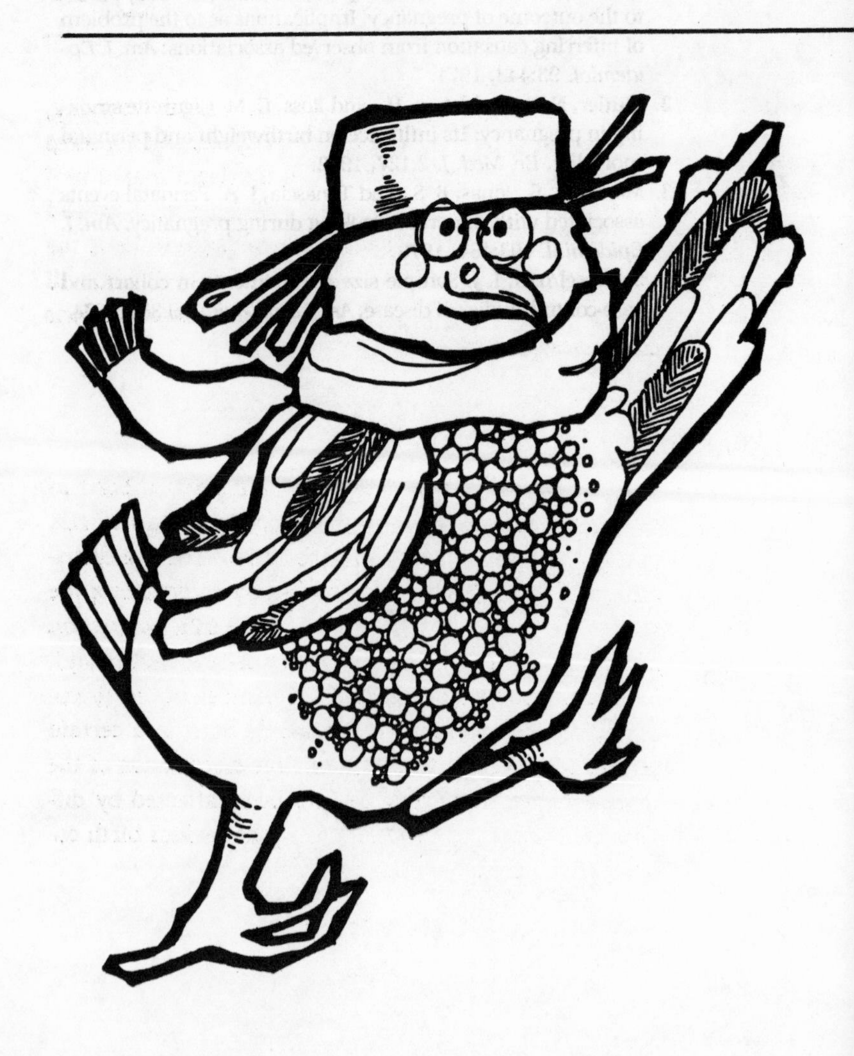

11. Cohort Effect

The Cohort Effect lives for the moment, never worrying, and hardly ever thinking, about the vagaries and concerns of the past. While his unbridled enthusiasm makes him a winning companion, his impulsive character can lead you into trouble. Thinking only of the present, he is the quintessential Gatsby, a rollicking ne'er-do-well who will show you some fun. Look for him in the halls and salons of cross-sectional research.

DEFINITION

The Cohort Effect is the tendency for persons born in certain years to carry a relatively higher (or lower) risk of a given disease throughout their lives. The age distribution of a disease is often studied by ascertaining the rate of the disease at one point in time in a population of widely varied age (a so-called cross-sectional study). Such a population will contain a number of "birth cohorts," which are made up of people born in a certain year or set of years. The apparent age distribution of the disease under study may be spuriously affected by differences in past experiences among the various birth cohorts in the study population.

CASE STUDY
Hemorrhoids at Devil's Piles, Wyoming

Conventional medical wisdom regarding the epidemiology, diagnosis, and therapy of hemorrhoids has been dominated for decades by the comprehensive work published by Dr. John Hindbeck in 1935, entitled *Grapes of Wrath: A Rational Approach to the Hemorrhoid.* A now classic study reviewed in Dr. Hindbeck's book was the survey of hemorrhoidal morbidity conducted in 1934 at Devil's Piles, Wyoming, by Drs. Stanley Itch and Sally Burns.

Drs. Itch and Burns carried out an extensive proctologic survey of 1,000 representative residents of Devil's Piles. Among their findings were the data shown in Table 13. Clearly apparent was a direct, stepwise increase in the prevalence of hemorrhoids with increasing age. Based on these findings, Itch and Burns speculated that the underlying etiology of hemorrhoids was a breakdown in vascular wall collagen concomitant with the overall aging process. This speculation led to the fashionable use of topical vitamin C for the treatment of hemorrhoids in the 1930s.

Comment

MacMahon and Pugh [1] have pointed out that at least three factors can affect the rate of a disease in a particular age group at a given point in time:

1. Factors characteristic of persons in the age group, because of their age *per se*
2. Factors characteristic of the *times* (for example, an epidemic that attacks different age groups with different intensity)
3. Past experiences of the birth cohorts that make up the various age groups at the time of the study

Table 13. Age-specific prevalence of hemorrhoids among residents of Devil's Piles (1934)

Age (yr)	Hemorrhoid cases per 100 residents
0–9	7
10–19	25
20–29	39
30–39	44
40–49	52
50–59	65

There is a natural tendency to infer that differences in disease rates found among people of different ages are due primarily to the *first* of these three factors. That is, we tend to conclude prematurely that if hemorrhoids are more prevalent in older folks, then something about *aging* causes hemorrhoids to occur. Watch your step! You are looking into the lively eyes of the Cohort Effect.

By 1940, a canny epidemiologist by the name of Dr. Beatrice Bottoms began to recognize that there were problems in the work of Itch and Burns. Bottoms was aware that horseback riding was a common means of transportation in Devil's Piles, and she began to think about the possibility that exposure to riding was etiologically important in the varying rates of hemorrhoids among different subgroups of the community's population. By exhaustively reviewing the medical records of the town doctor, Dr. Bottoms was able to compile a record of hemorrhoid incidence by increasing age for each of several birth cohorts, beginning with those born between 1880 and 1890 (Table 14).

Notice that, contrary to the conclusions of Drs. Itch and Burns, there is a gradual *decrease* in hemorrhoid diagnoses with increasing age, within each of the five birth cohorts studied. How can we account for the opposing findings of the two studies?

The 1934 cross-sectional data of Drs. Itch and Burns is displayed in Figure 8 as a solid line, with the birth cohort data of Bottoms shown in broken lines. It now is apparent that the cross-sectional study reached mistaken conclusions regarding the effect of aging on hemorrhoids. Within each age group, there is a gradual decrease in hemorrhoid prevalence over the years, *but starting from widely discrepant baselines.*

Through interviews with members of the various birth cohorts, Dr. Bottoms was able to confirm a gradual decrease in childhood exposure to horseback riding over the years, accounting for the successive downward shifts in hemorrhoid prevalence. Thus, the 1920 cohort differed

Table 14. Prevalence of hemorrhoids with increasing age among birth cohorts in Devil's Piles

Birth cohort	Hemorrhoid cases per 100 residents					
	0–9 yr	10–19 yr	20–29 yr	30–39 yr	40–49 yr	50–59 yr
1880–1890	80	75	73	71	68	65
1890–1900	67	61	58	55	52	
1900–1910	51	49	46	44		
1910–1920	46	42	39			
1920–1930	33	25				

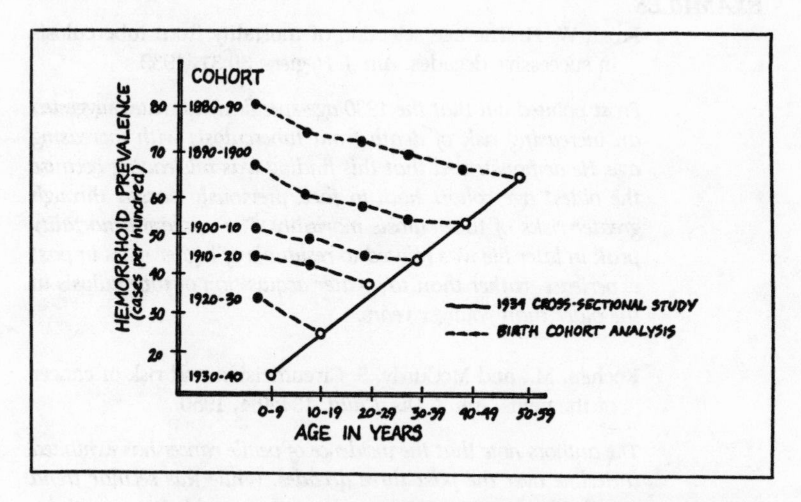

Figure 8. Hemorrhoid incidence by age: Comparison of cross-sectional study with birth cohort analysis.

from the 1880 cohort primarily in its greater use of carts, wagons, and automobiles, when cars emerged as an alternative form of transportation. In 1934, the 50- to 59-year-old age group had more hemorrhoids, not because aging begets hemorrhoids, but because they had *started* with a higher prevalence as a result of sitting on horses.

Drs. Itch and Burns were swept away by the Cohort Effect and blinded by his merry ways. Never forget to pause for a moment and contemplate the past when you are in the vicinity of cross-sectional research.

EXAMPLES

Frost, W. H. The age selection of mortality from tuberculosis in successive decades. *Am. J. Hygiene* 30:31, 1939.

Frost pointed out that the 1930 age-specific death rates suggested an increasing risk of death from tuberculosis with increasing age. He demonstrated that this finding was misleading because the oldest age cohort had, in fact, previously passed through greater risks of tuberculosis mortality. The apparent mortality peak in later life was related to residuals of higher rates in past experience, rather than to greater acquisition of tuberculosis in the older than younger years.

Kochen, M., and McCurdy, S. Circumcision and risk of cancer of the penis. *Am. J. Dis. Child.* 134:484, 1980.

The authors note that the incidence of penile cancer has exhibited a decline over the past three decades. While this secular trend may be due in part to improved economic and living conditions, it could also be related to a cohort effect. Increased circumcision rates in younger cohorts may have contributed to the overall lowering of penile cancer incidence in the entire population.

Levin, M. L. The occurrence of lung cancer in man. *Acta Unio Internationalis Contra Cancrum* 9:531, 1953.

This is an example of birth cohort analysis in the study of lung cancer mortality.

Susser, M. Period effects, generation effects and age effects in peptic ulcer mortality. *J. Chronic Dis.* 35:29, 1982.

This paper addresses the cohort effect in the context of peptic ulcer mortality for England and Wales, from 1900 to 1977.

SUGGESTED READING

Lilienfeld, A. M., and Lilienfeld, D. E. *Foundations of Epidemiology.* New York: Oxford University Press, 1980. Pp. 117–122.

The Lilienfelds' book is a useful primer of epidemiology and contains a good section on cohort effects.

REFERENCE

1. MacMahon, B., and Pugh, T. F. *Epidemiology: Principles and Methods.* Boston: Little, Brown, 1970. Pp. 184-198.

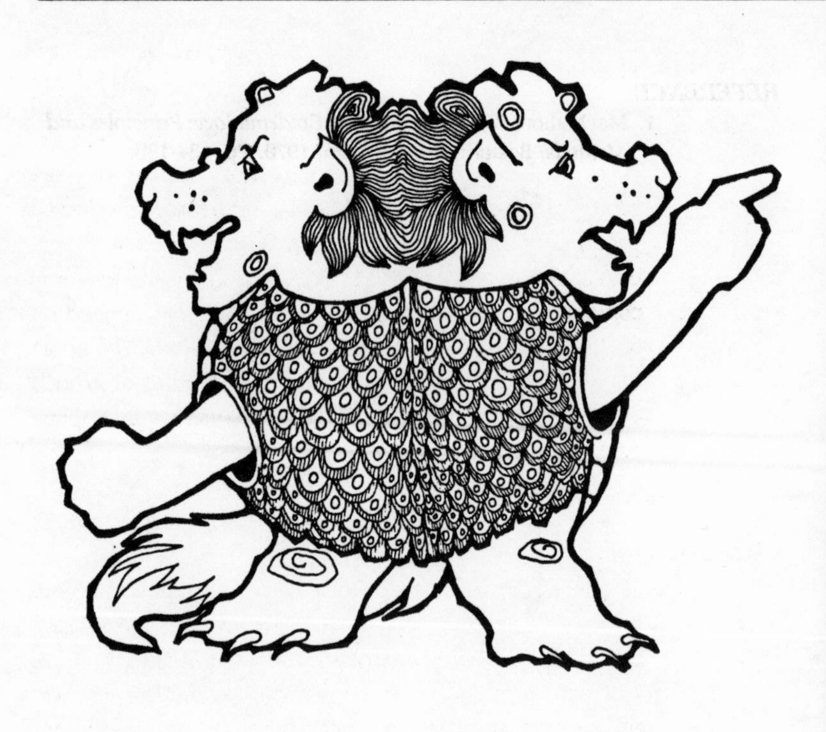

12. Ecologic Fallacy

The Ecologic Fallacy is a foxy, two-faced beast who lurks in the darkened corners of large population studies and tricks unwary readers into accepting unwarranted conclusions. This fellow can often be found infesting so-called ecologic research, in which *groups* of people in selected geographic areas, census tracts, or other specified locations are the units of study. Crafty and sly, he presents conclusions that may be valid or may be false, depending on the mouth from which he chooses to speak. To abort his trickery, you must remember that studies of groups can lead to spurious conclusions when uncritically applied to individuals.

DEFINITION

The Ecologic Fallacy is a mistaken conclusion that can be reached when one infers the behavior or experience of individuals from the behavior or experience of groups. While inferences from groups to individuals are often a useful stage in hypothesis development, the fallacy arises when it is *assumed* that an association observed in groups also occurs in individuals. This fallacy is most common in large, cross-sectional studies that examine epidemiologic characteristics of people in certain census tracts, counties, or other geographically defined areas.

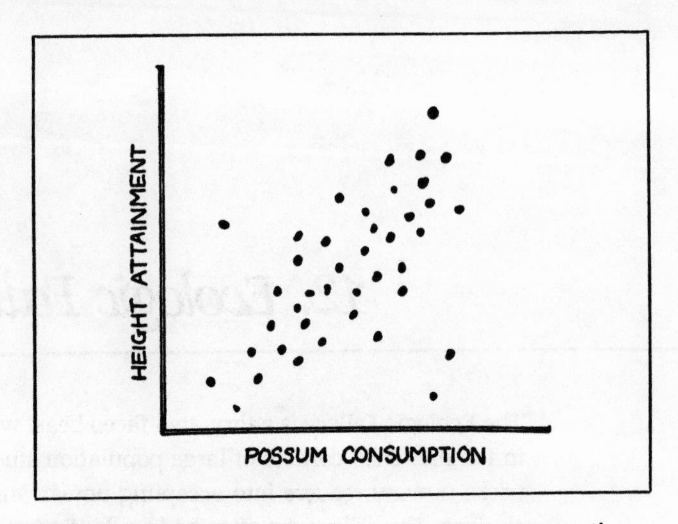

Figure 9. North Carolina county mean possum consumption by height attainment.

CASE STUDY
Possum Consumption and Growth

Reporting in the *Appalachian Journal of Nutritional Statistics*, Drs. Chu and Swallow examined the contribution of dietary possum to physical growth during the first five years of life. A random sample of families was used to estimate the average family's possum consumption in each of the 100 North Carolina counties. In addition, school records in each county were reviewed to ascertain mean height attainment for all five year olds residing in that county. Each county received two scores: average family possum consumption and average height at five years of age. Analysis of these data (Fig. 9) showed a strong positive association between height attainment and possum consumption, suggesting that utilization of possum as a dietary source of protein may have important, beneficial effects on growth in early childhood.

Comment

Data on the behavior or experience of groups can sometimes produce unreliable conclusions about the behavior or experience of individuals. Data about individuals are therefore almost always more useful than group data. However, group data are frequently more accessible. The Census Bureau, for example, aggregates data by census tract, and states usually summarize data by counties. It is generally cheaper and faster to use the existing group data in testing specific hypotheses. In such studies, the relationship of interest is still the possible association between some risk factor and a change in the health of an individual, but the association is evaluated using only the average rates for a collection of *groups*, not descriptive data on a collection of individuals. When conclusions are then offered about the risk of disease among individuals, beware: the beast of ecologic fallacies is smiling a toothy smile.

In the case of possum-eating and growth, the doctors'

conclusion that increasing dietary possum may improve growth in preschool children was a conclusion about individual children derived from data on county means. However, since the documented association was between county averages and not based on measurements of individual children, the results must be interpreted warily.

The fallacy in Chu and Swallow's ecologic study is demonstrated in subsequent work in which the observed association was tested on a random sample of children within each of three counties (Fig. 10). While the county averages suggest a strong positive association between possum consumption and height, individual data from within each county showed no such relationship.

How were we fooled by the original study? As shown in Figure 10, mountain counties tended to have both low average heights and low possum consumption, while coastal counties tended to have *high* means for both variables. The combination of these county characteristics resulted in the tentative (and wrong) conclusion that possum-eating results in improved growth. In fact, the apparent relationship resulted from other county characteristics that were not taken into consideration: namely, that possums were scarce in mountain counties and that mountain county residents were largely members of a low socioeconomic class (whose children tended to be smaller in height), while coastal counties had plenty of possums and higher social classes.

A good, nonfictitious example of the ecologic fallacy is the observed association between tuberculosis and crowding, as determined by census tract data. The relationship turns out to be a secondary association created by the confounding relationship of both crowding and tuberculosis to socioeconomic status. In fact, individuals with tuberculosis are most likely to be living alone, surrounded by households in which a large number of people live in a relatively small space.

Watch for the Ecologic Fallacy! He is always around when populations of people are the unit of study, and

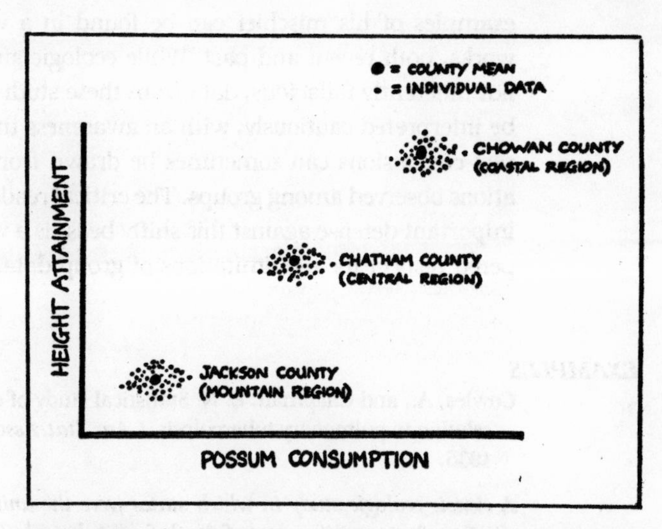

Figure 10. Individual data on possum consumption by height attainment.

examples of his mischief can be found in a variety of works, both recent and past. While ecologic studies are not inherently fallacious, data from these studies should be interpreted cautiously, with an awareness that incorrect conclusions can sometimes be drawn from associations observed among groups. The critical reader's most important defense against this shifty beast is a well-tempered respect for the limitations of group data.

EXAMPLES

Cowles, A., and Chapman, E. N. Statistical study of climate in relation to pulmonary tuberculosis. *J. Am. Stat. Assoc.* 30:517, 1935.

A classic ecologic study in which states were the unit of investigation. State-specific rates of death from tuberculosis were examined in relation to a variety of factors describing ecologic characteristics of the individual states. One finding was that hours of sunshine and altitude were inversely related to tuberculosis mortality.

Dodge, D. L., and Martin, W. T. *Social Stress and Chronic Illness.* South Bend, IN: University of Notre Dame Press, 1970.

Using data on state populations, the authors demonstrate an inverse relationship between social status inconsistency (that is, inconsistencies among social status hierarchies such as education, income, and occupation) and chronic disease rates. This is an example of an ecologic correlation that has been substantiated in studies of individuals.

Ober, W. B. Testimony given before the House of Representatives Committee on Interstate and Foreign Commerce, 1969.

Ober is quoted in an American Tobacco Company pamphlet as having testified that "there are certain well-known data which the cigarette-lung cancer hypothesis does not explain. For example, in Great Britain the per capita consumption of cigarettes is half as much as in the United States but the incidence of lung cancer is twice as much." It does not follow from this ecologic observation that lung cancer is not a potential consequence of smoking. In fact, the weight of evidence is clearly in favor of such a link, despite ecologic observations to the contrary.

Robinson, W. S. Ecological correlations and the behavior of individuals. *Am. Sociol. Rev.* 15:351, 1950.

Robinson noted that there is a moderate positive association in the United States between being foreign-born and being illiterate. However, when studied in terms of geographic regions, the same variables are negatively correlated.

SUGGESTED READING

Morgenstern, H. Uses of ecologic analysis in epidemiologic research. *Am. J. Public Health* 72:1336, 1982.

This is a comprehensive discussion of the uses and abuses of ecologic studies.

Thorndike, E. L. On the fallacy of imputing the correlations found for groups to the individuals or smaller groups composing them. *Am. J. Psychol.* 52:122, 1939.

Using individual and group data on the correlation between IQ and residential crowding, Thorndike demonstrated the mathematical basis for the ecologic fallacy.

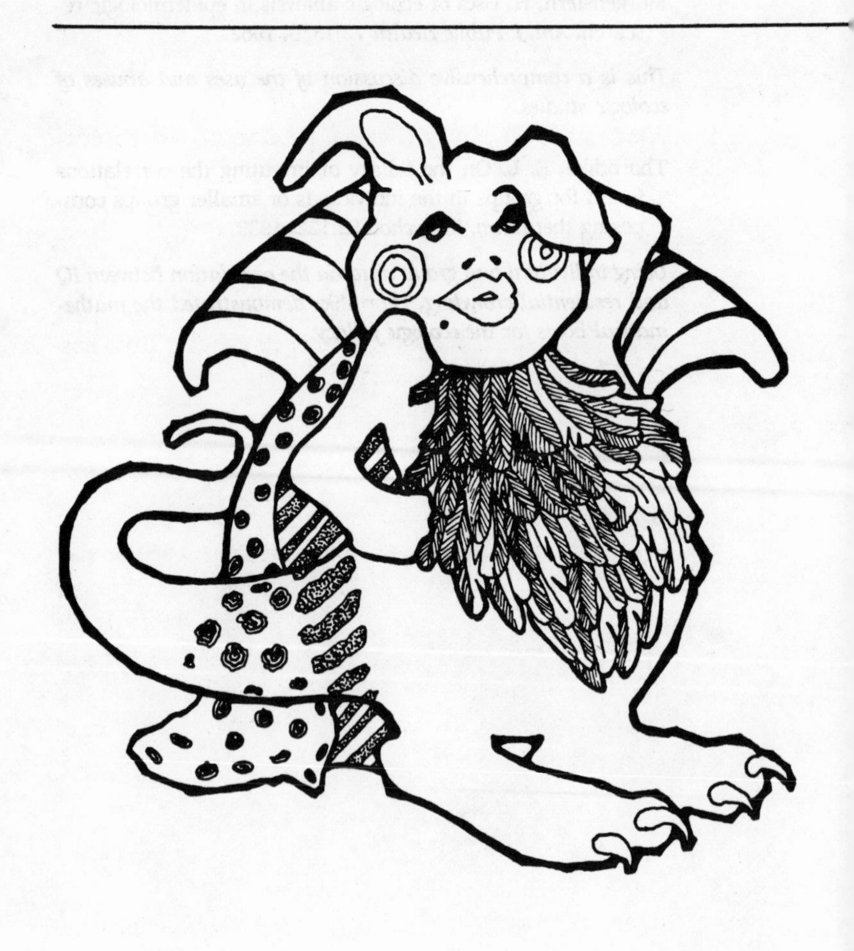

13. Berkson Bias

The Berkson Bias is a charmer, the Scarlett O'Hara of case-control studies. By changing her moods, her scents, her songs, and her style she selectively attracts people into a hospital or clinic. Her influence on who uses the hospital or clinic in a case-control study can result in spurious findings. Our Berkson Bias is elusive and difficult to capture. Nonetheless, echoes of her siren call waft over every case-control study that draws its subjects from hospital or clinic patient groups.

DEFINITION

Researchers conducting case-control studies of patients drawn from a clinic or hospital may arrive at false conclusions when the combination of disease and exposure are over-represented or under-represented in the study population. This distortion may be due to the type of hospital, the special interests of the medical staff, the nature of the medical problem, or the characteristics of the patients.

CASE STUDY

Is Diabetes Mellitus Caused By the Wart Virus?

Intensive research continues to suggest a viral etiology of juvenile-onset diabetes mellitus. Isolated case reports strongly support this claim and animal models add credibility to the viral hypothesis. Missing, however, is an acceptable biochemical or clinical marker of this viral infection that would permit the hypothesis to be tested in epidemiologic studies.

Dr. Susan Sweetpea recently made a curious observation during her endocrinology fellowship at the world-famous International Health Center. Many of her juvenile-onset diabetic patients also had a long history of plantar warts. Prompted by the earlier reports of a possible viral etiology of diabetes, Dr. Sweetpea hypothesized that warts might be a marker of that viral infection. In order to test this hypothesis she undertook a case-control study.

Medical records from 100 patients with juvenile-onset diabetes mellitus who were admitted to the International Health Center were randomly selected. For her comparison group she chose nondiabetic patients who were matched for age, sex, and race. Two controls for each diabetic case were selected.

All records were reviewed for mention of plantar warts. Table 15 shows the results of Dr. Sweetpea's study. Seventeen percent of the diabetic patients had had a history of warts, compared to 7.5 percent of the control patients. In other words, patients with diabetes were found to be more than twice as likely to have a history of warts as patients without diabetes.

Impressed with Dr. Sweetpea's findings, the International Health Center's Department of Medicine plans to extend these observations by carefully screening all hospital admissions for plantar warts. The Division of Infectious Diseases is concurrently evaluating serum samples on all admissions in an effort to elaborate the serologic changes associated with warts that may indicate the pathophysiologic link with juvenile-onset diabetes mellitus.

Comment

Case-control studies often use hospitals or clinics to identify patients, usually because of the ready access to the

Table 15. Juvenile-onset diabetes and plantar warts (International Health Center study)

Study group	With warts	Without warts	Total
Diabetics	17 (17%)	83 (83%)	100
Nondiabetics	15 (7.5%)	185 (92.5%)	200

medical records. However, patients identified in this way may not be entirely representative because of selective hospital or clinic utilization patterns related to the type of facility or patient characteristics.

Dr. Sweetpea found that a history of plantar warts was more common among hospitalized diabetic patients, which suggested that warts are related to the risk of juvenile-onset diabetes. Dr. Sweetpea chose her cases and controls carefully and had ample laboratory evidence to support the basic idea of a link between diabetes and warts. However, her diligence did not save her from the Berkson Bias.

Results of a larger community-based study sponsored by the Verruca Foundation did not confirm the original results. As shown in Table 16, 12.7 percent of diabetes patients had warts, compared to 13.6 percent of the controls. There was no identifiable risk for diabetes among sufferers of plantar warts.

Closer scrutiny of the health center's records revealed a possible reason Dr. Sweetpea's study had led to a spurious association. Adjacent to the hospital is a large podiatry clinic that refers all of its patients, many with diabetes, to the health center. The referral of these patients probably resulted in a selective over-representation of diabetics with plantar warts in the original hospital-based study. Other peculiarities of patient referral or physicians' interest could similarly affect Dr. Sweetpea's sample and consequent conclusions.

The association of pancreatitis and hyperparathyroidism is an interesting example of how the Berkson Bias can affect clinical thinking. In 1962, a large study suggested an association between pancreatitis and hyperparathyroidism [1]. This presumed causal association remained an accepted part of medical knowledge until a follow-up study was published in 1980 [2].

In the original study, the diagnosis of hyperparathyroidism and pancreatitis was made in hospitalized patients on clinical grounds. In the follow-up study the au-

Table 16. Juvenile-onset diabetes and plantar warts (Verruca Foundation study)

	With warts	Without warts	Total
Diabetics	96 (12.7%)	660 (87.3%)	756
Nondiabetics	3,030 (13.6%)	21,155 (86.4%)	24,185

thors point out that the diagnosis of hyperparathyroidism is now made biochemically through routine, outpatient screening and rarely leads to hospitalization, while the diagnosis and management of pancreatitis still entail hospitalization. The original study was biased because the hospital sample did not accurately reflect the prevalence of hyperparathyroidism.

The Berkson Bias can work her charms on any case-control study that is not population based—and very few are. Unfortunately, it's difficult to accurately predict how the events that lead to hospital or medical care utilization might result in this form of selection bias. The possibility of the Berkson Bias is simply another reason why a single epidemiologic study is seldom sufficient to prove an association. Confirmation of a finding by several different studies in several different populations greatly enhances the strength of any finding.

EXAMPLES

Gerber, L. M., Wolf, A. M., Braham, R. L., and Alderman, M. H. Effects of sample selection on the coincidence of hypertension and diabetes. *J.A.M.A.* 247:43, 1982.

In this study, the ability of Berkson Bias to alter the observed pattern of disease and thereby limit extrapolation of results to other populations is examined. Patients seen in a general, university-based medical clinic and in a work-site clinic setting showed different patterns of disease expression. Patients seen in the university-based general medical clinic had more strokes, heart attacks, and problems with diabetic control than did patients seen at the work-site clinic. The authors suggest that the conclusions of clinical studies drawn from university settings may not accurately reflect what is experienced in a community setting because of selective differences in the two patient groups. Thus, Berkson Bias could modify our understanding of the natural history of these diseases.

Meyer, C. T., Troncale, F. T., Galloway, S., et al. Arteriovenous malformations of the bowel. An analysis of 22 cases and a review of the literature. *Medicine* 60:36, 1981.

Williams, R. C. Aortic stenosis and unexplained gastrointestinal bleeding. *Arch. Intern. Med.* 108:103, 1961.

The association between aortic stenosis and intestinal arteriovenous malformations, first suggested by Williams, has fascinated and baffled clinicians for years. Several large series seemed to indicate a causal relationship, although the suggested pathophysiologic mechanisms were somewhat strained. In the review by Meyer and colleagues of the purported association it is pointed out that old people frequently acquire both conditions, and many episodes of occult gastrointestinal bleeding are caused by ectatic blood vessels that have no relationship to aortic stenosis.

Berkson, J. Limitations of the application of fourfold table analysis to hospital data. *Biometr. Bull.* 2:47, 1946.

This is the paper that started it all.

Brown, G. W. Berkson fallacy revisited. *Am. J. Dis. Child.* 130:56, 1976.

This is a discussion of the mathematics involved in the Berkson Bias, plus several examples.

Ibrahim, M. A. (Ed.). The case-control study: Consensus and controversy. *J. Chronic Dis.* 32:1–144, 1979.

The potential importance of Berkson Bias is debated by Drs. Feinstein, Sackett, and Vessey in this interesting collection of papers. Each expert expresses a different opinion of this epidemiologic hazard and the extent to which it is a serious disruptor of case-control studies.

REFERENCES

1. Mixter, C. G., Keyes, W. M., and Cope, O. Further experience with pancreatitis as a diagnostic clue to hyperparathyroidism. *N. Engl. J. Med.* 266:265, 1962.
2. Bess, M. A., Edis, A. J., and VanHeerden, J. A. Hyperparathyroidism and pancreatitis. *J.A.M.A.* 243:246, 1980.

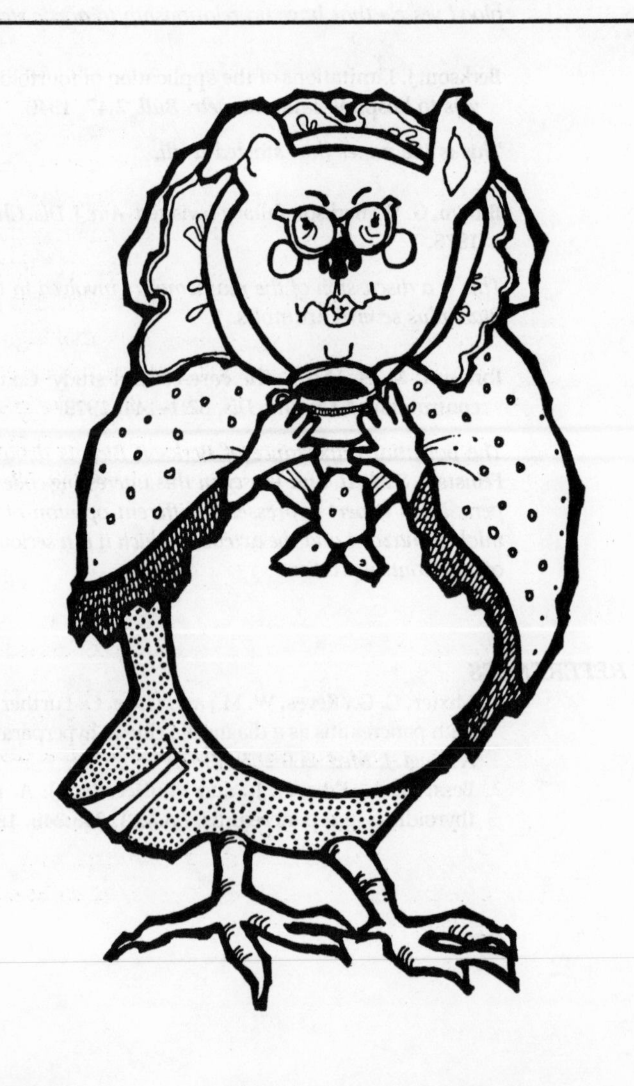

14. Matchmaker

The Matchmaker is an elderly aunt who has taken up permanent occupancy in the living rooms of case-control research. Unfortunately, she is never there when you really need her, but always there when you don't. She hovers over case-control studies like a matronly queen, whispering "have I got a control for you . . ." into the ear of the hapless investigator. The trick with this shrewd old bat is to use her as you need her, making careful and cautious decisions about your requirements for her matchmaking services. When reading, take great care that you are not lured into unhesitating acceptance of the mistaken conclusions of a study flawed by the Matchmaker.

DEFINITION

Under-matching is the failure to select cases and controls that are sufficiently alike in important characteristics. When under-matched, a case-control study can demonstrate a spurious association between a disease and a supposed cause.

Over-matching is the error of selecting controls that *excessively* resemble the cases. When over-matched, a case-control study can fail to discover an association that, in fact, is present and real.

Table 17. Speech patterns and malignant melanoma

		Speech pattern	
Study group	Number	Slow	Regular
Melanoma cases	1,000	730 (73%)	270 (27%)
Controls	1,000	450 (45%)	550 (55%)

$\chi^2 = 162$
$p < .001$

CASE STUDIES

Melanoma and Sweet Talk

In 1945, the Drs. Beauregard and Tate published a paper in the *South Georgia Medical Gazette* that claimed to demonstrate a strong association between certain speech patterns and malignant melanoma. A random sample of 1,000 adult males with melanoma was drawn from the tumor registries in each of the 50 states. The 1,000 control subjects were selected and matched with melanoma cases according to age, social class, and type of employment. Drs. Beauregard and Tate then carried out interviews with each of the 2,000 study participants. Interviews were designed to assess a wide range of personal, life-style, and job characteristics for the case and control populations.

Analysis of the data (Table 17) indicated that the greatest difference between cases and controls was the disproportionate number of cases who spoke in the characteristic, slow cadenced, long-voweled pattern of speech known as a southern drawl. Seventy-three percent of patients with melanoma were slow talkers, as compared to 45 percent of the control group ($p < .001$).

Beauregard and Tate's study led to the now infamous Speech Act of 1948 mandating a national melanoma prevention program, which provided speech therapy for all citizens noted on simple screening test to utilize the contraction "y'all."

Chronic Bronchitis and Air Pollution

Drs. Hack and Koff recently reported the results of a study that has left the world of pulmonary medicine gasping for breath. Speaking before the annual meeting of the London Phlegm Society, they called into question the widely accepted relationship between air pollution and chronic bronchitis.

Utilizing a case-control design, 100 adults with a diagnosis of chronic bronchitis were identified in the greater

New York metropolitan area. For each patient with bronchitis, a control person was selected who lived in the same census tract (to assure comparability in social class) and who matched the patient with respect to age, sex, race, and smoking status. Cases and controls were then compared on a variety of environmental and health behavioral dimensions.

Among the important results of the study was the finding that exposure to polluted air was identical in the case and control groups. The average neighborhood pollution level for both groups was 82 mg/m^3. This startling discovery will undoubtedly be used to justify deregulation of industries that generate atmospheric pollutants.

Comments

Case-control studies are often used to explore a new hypothesis about the relationship between a disease and its suspected cause. Such studies begin by identifying persons with the disease (the cases) and comparing them to a second group of persons who do not have the disease (the controls) in order to ascertain differences in the degree of exposure to the hypothesized cause. Because case-control studies begin after the diagnosis has already been made and look backwards (or retrospectively) at possible causes, the cost and complexity of such a study is relatively low.

One of the potential pitfalls of case-control research is the way control subjects are chosen. Most diseases have many factors that contribute to the risk of their occurrence. The risk of lung cancer, for example, is enhanced by smoking, increasing age, male sex, and exposure to environmental factors such as asbestos. The purpose of *matching* controls to certain known characteristics of the cases is to ensure that cases and controls have approximately equal susceptibility to the disease in terms of all risk factors except the one in question. It is here that the elderly Matchmaker may lure and embarrass the less than vigilant researcher.

It is often difficult to know which factors are important to match. Furthermore, the process of matching controls to cases can be extremely costly, in terms of both money and time. In general, cases and controls are matched for the risk factors that are most strongly related to both the exposure and the disease (Fig. 11). For example, in a study of smoking years and lung cancer, controls should be matched with cases according to age since any association found might be partly due to the confounding effect of age on both smoking years and cancer.

Under-matching may occur when important confounding factors are not accounted for in the matching process. When under-matched, a case-control study can demonstrate strong associations that are invalid because of the underlying effect of an uncontrolled risk factor. However, there are analytical and statistical methods that can be used at the conclusion of a study to control for the confounding effects of unmatched variables, given that data on those variables have been collected. Thus, matching is not the only alternative in controlling for the effects of secondary risk factors.

Case-control studies can also be over-matched. Risk factors that are related only to the exposure and not to the disease (Fig. 12) should not be matched. Over-matching tends to make differences in the exposure rate less apparent, even when the differences are present. The real differences in exposures are "diluted out" by controlling for the confounding factor. Watch how the studies were flawed by under- or over-matching in our analysis of the case studies; each of our investigators was tricked by the guile of Madam Matchmaker.

Drs. Beauregard and Tate made the mistake of forgetting to match on a crucial risk factor that was related to both the exposure (slow talk) and the disease (melanoma). Exposure to high levels of sunlight is a charac-

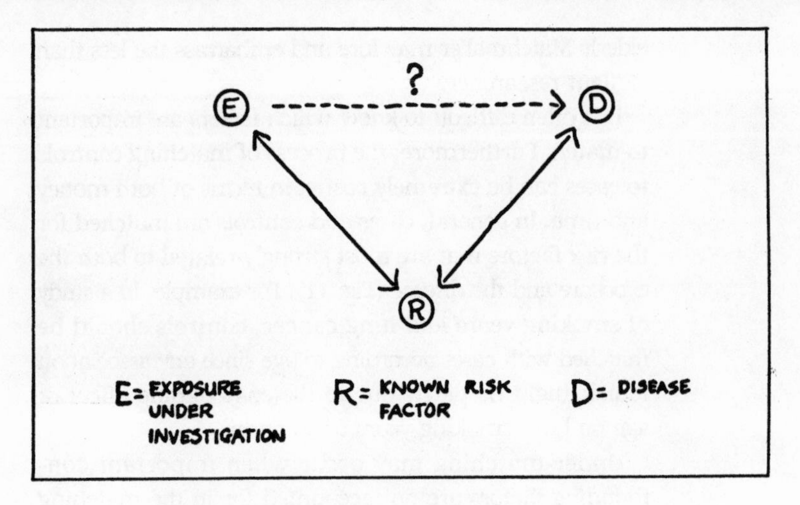

Figure 11. Relationships among exposure, risk factors, and disease in case-control studies.

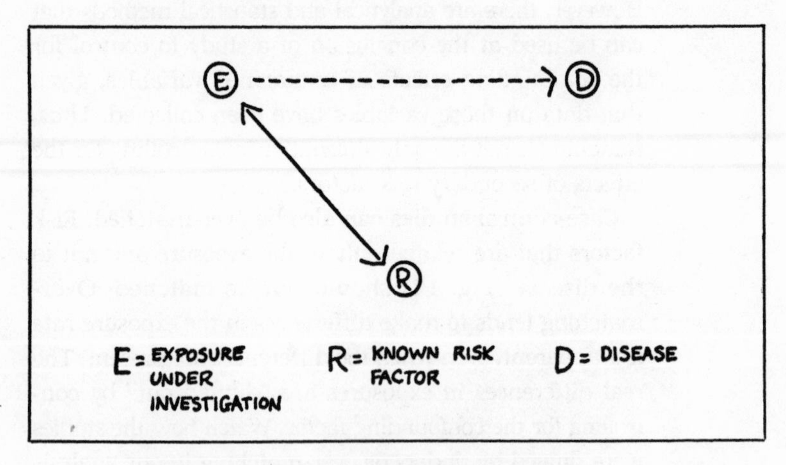

Figure 12. Relationships among exposure, risk factors, and disease in an over-matched case-control study.

Table 18. Speech patterns and malignant melanoma, controlling for geographic area

		Speech pattern	
Study group	Number	Slow	Regular
Northern U.S.			
Melanoma cases	100	10 (10%)	90 (90%)
Controls	500	50 (10%)	450 (90%)
Southern U.S.			
Melanoma cases	900	720 (80%)	180 (20%)
Controls	500	400 (80%)	100 (20%)

$$\text{Overall case drawl rate} = \frac{10 + 720}{1{,}000} = 73\%$$

$$\text{Overall control drawl rate} = \frac{50 + 400}{1{,}000} = 45\%$$

$\chi^2 = 0$, p = not significant

teristic common to both people who speak with a drawl and people who have melanoma. The relationship between southern speech patterns and melanoma can be fully accounted for by the confounding effect of sunlight exposure. Table 18 reconstructs the error of Beauregard and Tate's ways by analyzing according to geographical area. Table 18 demonstrates that when cases and controls who are drawn from the same region are compared, no differences in drawl rates are found. (This method of separating the study population into groups in order to remove the effect of a confounder is called stratification.) Healthy controls in the original study showed a relatively low drawl rate because they were drawn in approximately equal numbers from northern and southern areas. Melanoma cases, on the other hand, were identified primarily in the southern states, where both high levels of solar radiation and high drawl rates are found together. Drs. Beauregard and Tate would have reached the correct conclusion (i.e., that there is *no* relationship between slow talk and melanoma) if they had taken into account the degree of exposure to sunlight by matching cases to controls according to geographic area.

In the second case study, Drs. Hack and Koff erred by inadvertently matching for the very factor they were investigating as a cause of bronchitis. By choosing their controls from the same census tracts in which the cases lived, they matched according to the neighborhood of residence. Since the neighborhood is related to the exposure (air pollution), it was impossible for their cases and controls to differ in exposure to air pollution. This over-match renders the association between pollution and bronchitis invisible. Table 19 presents the data from their study. The last column shows the difference in results when a new set of controls was not matched with cases by neighborhood, but instead chosen randomly from all London neighborhoods: Air pollution exposure is now seen to be markedly less in controls than cases. By choosing controls who lived in the same neighborhood as the

Table 19. Comparison of average pollution exposure of bronchitis patients, controls matched by neighborhood, and controls not matched by neighborhood

Study group	No. from high-pollution neighborhood (100 mg/m^3)	No. from low-pollution neighborhood (10 mg/m^3)	Average pollution exposure
Bronchitis patients	80	20	82 mg/m^3 [a]
Controls			
Matched by neighborhood	80	20	82 mg/m^3 [b]
Not matched by neighborhood	50	50	55 mg/m^3 [c]

[a] Average case pollution $= \frac{(80 \times 100) + (20 \times 10)}{100} = 82\ mg/m^3$

[b] Average control (matched by neighborhood) pollution $= \frac{(80 \times 100) + (20 \times 10)}{100} = 82\ mg/m^3$

[c] Average control (not matched by neighborhood) pollution $= \frac{(50 \times 100) + (50 \times 10)}{100} = 55\ mg/m^3$

cases, the investigators eliminated any possibility of demonstrating the differences in air pollution exposure among persons with and without bronchitis.

Go cautiously into the territory of case-control research! Matching is an extraordinarily difficult job, and there is usually no simple answer to the questions of how to match, or whether to match at all. Significant associations may change with strategic changes in the character of the match. Behind it all is the large, imperious Matchmaker, always on hand to convince you that she has picked just the right control. Don't agree to anything until you see who she has in mind!

EXAMPLES

Bross, J. D. J. How case-for-case matching can improve design efficiency. *Am. J. Epidemiol.* 89:359, 1969.

This paper discusses a typical example of the problem of confounding in case-control studies. The author examines the confounding role of age in an exploration of an etiologic relationship between lactation and breast cancer. Since age is a factor related to both the exposure and the disease, matching in this situation will decrease the probability of finding an invalid association.

Starko, K. M., Ray, C. G., Dominguez, L. B., et al. Reye's syndrome and salicylate use. *Pediatrics* 66:859, 1980.

Waldman, R. J., Hall, W. N., McGee, H., et al. Aspirin as a risk factor in Reye's syndrome. *J.A.M.A.* 247:3089, 1982.

Halpin, T. J., Holtzhauer, F. J., Campbell, R. J., et al. Reye's syndrome and medication use. *J.A.M.A.* 248:687, 1982.

For a current example of the difficulty surrounding proper selection of matched controls, see this set of papers on the relationship of salicylate ingestion to Reye's syndrome. Reye's syndrome is known to follow certain viral illnesses, such as influenza and chickenpox in children, and salicylate use is more common among individuals experiencing such illnesses. Viral illness therefore constitutes an important confounding risk factor in the association between salicylate use and Reye's syndrome. Part of the controversy that followed these reports thus dealt with the appropriateness of the case-control match according to the type of preceding illness. Also note, in the paper by Halpin and associates, the use of statistical *methods to control for confounders as an alternative to matching.*

SUGGESTED READING

Gullen, W. H. A danger in matched-control studies. *J.A.M.A.* 224:2279, 1980.

Over-matching is discussed in this paper.

Hayden, G. F., Kramer, M. S., and Horwitz, R. I. The case-control study: A practical review for the clinician. *J.A.M.A.* 247:326, 1982.

A review of the case-control study as a research design—written by and for clinicians.

Horwitz, R. I., and Feinstein, A. R. Methodologic standards and contradictory results in case-control research. *Am. J. Med.* 66:556, 1979.

This paper summarizes the difficulties inherent in case-control research.

Ibrahim, M. A. (Ed.). The case-control study: Consensus and controversy. *J. Chronic Dis.* 32:1—144, 1979.

The entire issue of this journal was devoted to case-control research, its potential flaws and biases, and the development of methodological standards for evaluating such studies. This is a readable approach to the problems of case-control designs and includes various opinions about what makes a good match.

Miettinen, O. S. Matching and design efficiency in retrospective studies. *Am. J. Epidemiol.* 91:111, 1970.

This is a biostatistical, but understandable, discussion of the theoretical issues behind matching.

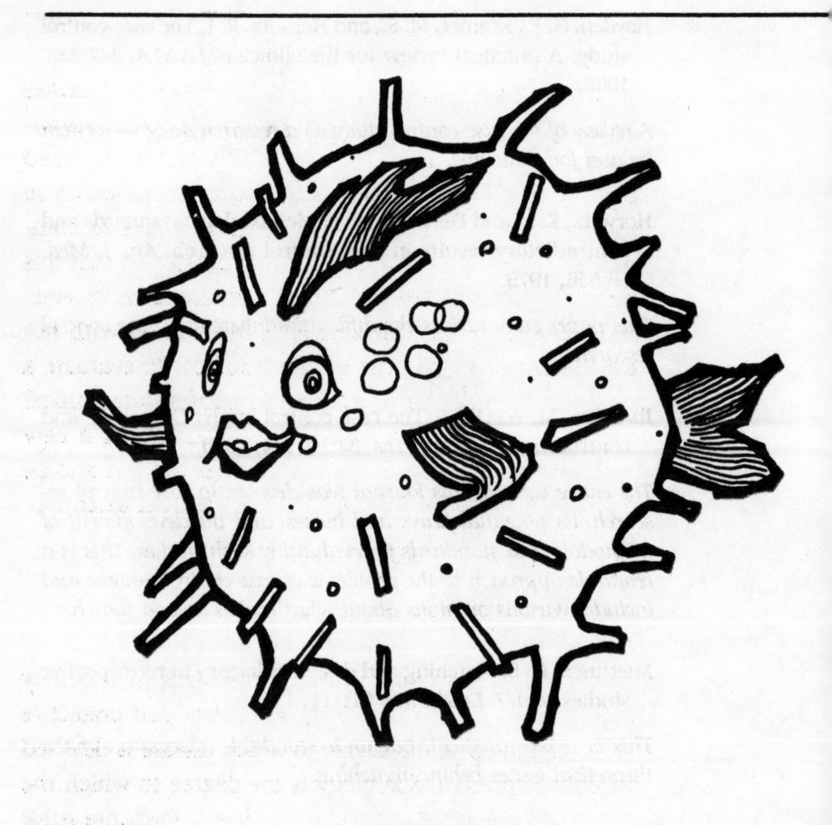

15. Test Bloater

It is his constant infatuation with new tests that makes the Test Bloater seem so silly at times. His boundless enthusiasm for first reports about a new test is mirrored by an improbable physique. As his excitement grows so too does the Test Bloater. He swells to a size of commanding importance, inflated by the conviction that this newest test offers the most useful measurements ever. As it happens, the Test Bloater is often filled with hot air. He has precious little insight into how to evaluate a new test in order to determine its appropriate clinical use. When confronted with his harangue about a new test, it is next to impossible not to order the test and be done with him. The Test Bloater may attract attention, but he usually ends up being a windbag.

DEFINITION

The usefulness of a new diagnostic test is determined by at least three criteria: sensitivity, specificity, and predictive value. *Sensitivity* is the degree to which disease is detected when it is present. *Specificity* is the degree to which the test is negative when the disease is absent. *Predictive value* is the degree to which a given test result is correct. One can measure the positive or negative predictive value of a test. Positive predictive value is the proportion of individuals with positive tests in whom the disease is actually present. Negative predictive value is the proportion of individuals with negative tests in whom no disease is found. The predictive value of a test depends not only on sensitivity and specificity but on the prevalence of the disease in the population being tested. Thus, the greater the prevalence, the higher the positive predictive value.

New tests are often tried out on groups of patients in which there is a high prevalence of the condition under study. Generally, the predictive value of the test under such conditions is much higher than under more usual clinical situations. Accordingly, the initial assessment of the predictive value of a test is often overly optimistic, even when the sensitivity and specificity are exactly known.

CASE STUDY
Serum Rhubarb Levels in the Diagnosis of Deep Venous Thrombosis

Researchers at the Berlin Institut des Blut recently revealed the discovery of a new test for the accurate diagnosis of deep venous thrombosis. This potentially life threatening condition, once suspected, is diagnosed correctly only half the time by clinical examination. The sine qua non of diagnosis has remained venography, which itself carries certain risks.

This new test uses an extract of rhubarb, in combination with washed blood cells from the domesticated cockroach, that when mixed with a patient's serum gives a distinctive slide precipitation pattern.

To examine the usefulness of the serum rhubarb test in actual clinical situations the institute initiated a study with the Central Hospital's Department of Radiology. The institute's researchers collaborated with Dr. Venus Klott II, the renowned radiologist at Central Hospital who has 35 years' experience doing venograms and whose extensive venography experience warrants referrals from the surrounding area. During a six-month study period Dr. Klott personally did venograms in all patients referred for sus-

Table 20. Serum rhubarb test in patients with suspected deep venous thrombosis

Results of rhubarb test	Deep venous thrombosis		
	Present	Absent	
Positive	62	4	66
Negative	6	53	59
	68	57	125

Sensitivity = 62/68 = 91%
Specificity = 53/57 = 93%
Positive predictive value = 62/66 = 94%

pected deep venous thrombosis. Sera from these patients were drawn for the serum rhubarb test; the results were made available to Dr. Klott after the venograms were completed and interpreted. During the six-month study period 125 patients were referred for venograms.

Table 20 shows the results of the serum rhubarb test in these 125 patients. Deep venous thrombosis was detected in 68 patients, of whom 62 had a positive test. Of the 57 patients with a negative venogram, 53 had a negative rhubarb test.

Based on these data, the serum rhubarb test has a sensitivity of 91 percent, a specificity of 93 percent, and a positive predictive value of 94 percent. Researchers and clinicians alike were pleased with these results. They concluded that the serum rhubarb test is a powerful and simple diagnostic tool for patients with suspected deep venous thrombosis, and they predicted that the test would dramatically reduce the need for the more invasive venogram. Its use in a variety of clinical settings should increase efficiency of patient management and dramatically improve patient outcomes. The results of this study will be published in the *Blutundgutsannals*.

Comment

Positive (and negative) predictive values are usually more useful than sensitivity and specificity to clinicians since these values indicate the "predictiveness" of a given test result in an individual patient. The results of the serum rhubarb test would seem to indicate a very useful test.

Following this research project, interns on the hospital medical and surgical services began to use the test routinely on patients they suspected of having deep venous thrombosis. After another six months of routine use, a review of the data showed quite unexpectedly that the positive predictive value had fallen from 94 percent to 68 percent (Table 21). The sensitivity and specificity of the test remained virtually unchanged at 92 percent and 93 percent, respectively. What was the problem?

Table 21. Serum rhubarb test results after six months routine use

Results of rhubarb test	Deep venous thrombosis		
	Present	Absent	
Positive	67	32	99
Negative	6	425	431
	73	457	530

Sensitivity = 67/73 = 92%

Specificity = 425/457 = 93%

Positive predictive value = 67/99 = 68%

Table 22. Criteria for evaluating the usefulness of a new diagnostic test

Diagnostic Test	Disease		
	Present	Absent	
Positive	a	b	(a+b)
Negative	c	d	(c+d)
	(a+c)	(b+d)	(a+b+c+d)

Sensitivity = likelihood of a positive test in patients with the disease $= \frac{a}{a+c}$

Specificity = likelihood of a negative test in patients without the disease $= \frac{d}{b+d}$

Positive predictive value = likelihood that a patient with a positive test actually has the disease $= \frac{a}{a+b}$

Negative predictive value = likelihood that a patient with a negative test is healthy $= \frac{d}{c+d}$

Sensitivity and specificity reflect the proportion of positive and negative test results in homogeneous populations of patients, that is, either those *with* the disease (for sensitivity) or those *without* the disease (for specificity). These two criteria are therefore unaffected by the ratio of diseased to healthy patients. Predictive value, on the other hand, is strongly affected by the proportion of diseased patients (the prevalence) in the study population (Table 22).

The Test Bloater inflated the original predictive value of the serum rhubarb test by deriving initial results from a highly selected population. The researchers assumed that since the test's value had been confirmed by a very experienced clinician it would give a high quality benchmark to apply in other settings. In fact, the opposite was true.

Dr. Klott's reputation as a venographer meant that a group of patients for whom there was a greater than average suspicion of thrombosis was referred to him for study. Consequently, 54 percent (68/125) of his study subjects did indeed prove to have deep venous thrombosis. This high prevalence mathematically inflates the positive predictive value for the serum rhubarb test.

In the usual clinical setting the test did not fare as well. The interns suspected deep venous thrombosis in a larger number of persons, many more of whom did not have documented clots. The lower prevalence increased the number of false positives. Only 14 percent (73/530) of their patients proved to have deep venous thrombosis. The lower and more usual prevalence of the disease reduced the positive predictive value for the interns' group. In effect, the higher positive predictive value of the test in Dr. Klott's hands reflected the selective nature of his practice.

The Test Bloater fails to consider that the initial results of a new test are usually derived from a group of patients with a high disease prevalence. These are the very populations that can give an inflated positive predictive value.

To the clinician, the diagnostic value of a test is often best estimated by positive predictive values obtained in ordinary clinical settings. In addition, factors such as expense, simplicity, patient acceptability, and whether the test is used in series or parallel with other tests must moderate enthusiasm for a new test.

While that perfect test always eludes us, the Test Bloater is always finding it—again and again and again. Don't let yourself get caught up in his enthusiasm.

EXAMPLES

Khan, M. A., and Khan, M. K. Diagnostic value of HLA-B27 testing in analyzing spondylitis and Reiter's syndrome. *Ann. Intern. Med.* 96:70, 1982.

HLA-B27 is associated with several rheumatologic disorders and has a reasonable predictive value in referral settings. As the authors point out, however, its value is very limited in the usual clinical setting, where the prevalence of these disorders is very low. This article contains an excellent discussion of the effect of prevalence on predictive value.

Pozen, M. W., D'Agostino, R. B., Mitchell, J. B., et al. The usefulness of a predictive instrument to reduce inappropriate admissions to the coronary care unit. *Ann. Intern. Med.* 92:238, 1980.

A mathematical model was developed by the authors in an attempt to reduce admissions of patients with noncardiac chest pain to the coronary care unit. The diagnostic accuracy rate for admissions increased significantly. However, enthusiasm for this "test" must be tempered. The patients under study came to a well-known hospital because they had chest pain and therefore may not be representative of other clinical groups. How useful the model will be in other settings must be further studied before it is adopted into clinical practice.

Rogers, L. E., Lyon, G. M., and Porter, F. S. Spot test for vanillylmandelic acid and other guaiacols in urine of patients with neuroblastoma. *Am. J. Clin. Pathol.* 58:383, 1972.

This new diagnostic test had a positive predictive value of 90%. However, the study population had a neuroblastoma prevalence of 13/268 (4.85%), compared to the actual prevalence in the general population of 2–3/100,000 (0.0003%). Thus, as a screening test for neuroblastoma, the spot urine test had a recalculated positive predictive value of 0.5 percent.

Van Herte, A. J. (Moderator). The thyroid nodule. *Ann. Intern. Med.* 96:221, 1982.

This is a detailed review of the various diagnostic tests used to evaluate the thyroid nodule. Using data collected from publications throughout the world, the authors formulate a diagnostic strategy based on the sensitivity, specificity, and predictive values of the various tests.

Watson, R. A., and Tang, D. B. The predictive value of prostatic acid phosphatase as a screening test for prostatic cancer. *N. Engl. J. Med.* 303:497, 1980.

A previous article and its companion editorial in the same journal issue stimulated this spirited analysis of the Test Bloater. What at first had been thought to be a tool for mass screening for prostatic cancer is shown by the authors to be suitable only for high-risk groups. Regardless of a test's sensitivity or specificity, predictive value hinges on the prevalence of the disease in the population tested.

SUGGESTED READING

Griner, P. F., Mayerwski, R. J., Mushlin, A. L., and Greenland, P. Selection and interpretation of diagnostic tests and procedures: II. Principles of test interpretations. *Ann. Intern. Med.* 94:565, 1981.

This is a review of the principles of sensitivity, specificity, and predictive values.

Griner, P. F., Mayerwski, M. D., Mushlin, A. I., and Greenland, P. Selection and interpretation of diagnostic tests and procedures: III. Application of principles of test selection and interpretation. *Ann. Intern. Med.* 94:573, 1981.

In this paper a set of exercises is used to explore the relationships between sensitivity and specificity of a test and the clinical likelihood of disease. Tests for iron deficiency anemia, carcinoma of the breast, and cholelithiasis are among the examples used.

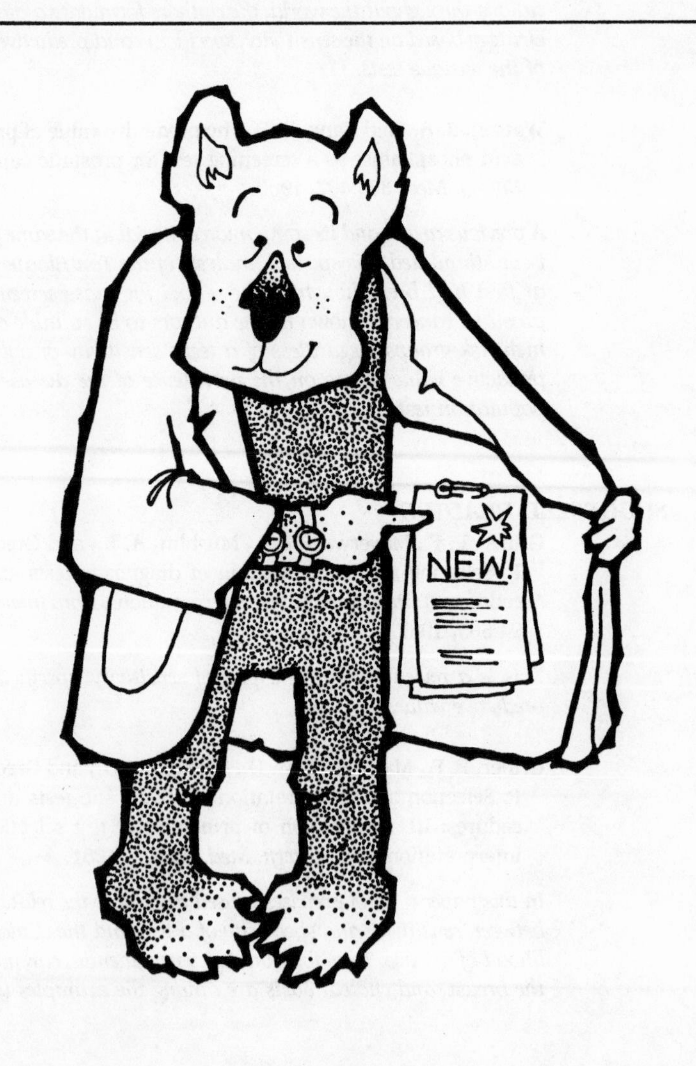
NEW!

16. Diagnostic Zealot

Above all, the Diagnostic Zealot is sincere. Evidence in hand, he stands before you as a humble and true believer, earnestly seeking your advocacy in the Diagnosis of Disease. For the most part, he is a peddler of the latest diagnostic test, proudly proclaiming its benefits and truths. By varying the intensity of the diagnostic workup or by skewing the clinical spectrum of patients, he has fooled himself (and may well fool you) into an unswerving belief in the benefits of a certain diagnostic test. Unlike many of his fellow fallacies, he is not a sinister chap. But be careful nonetheless! While his sincerity is alluring, his conclusions may be wrong.

DEFINITION

The efficacy of a diagnostic test may be spuriously inflated in at least two ways:

1. *Workup bias:* Conducting diagnostic workups of differing intensity in patients with differing test results
2. *Spectrum bias:* Evaluating the test in too narrow a clinical spectrum of disease

CASE STUDIES

Polka Dot Lung Disease

Screening with Nuclear Magnetic Resonance. In recent years much interest has focused on the use of nuclear magnetic resonance (NMR) in the diagnosis of certain occult diseases. In 1981, Dr. Susan Sleeper reported to the International Lung Congress about her work on the early detection of polka dot lung disease by use of NMR. Polka dot lung disease (PDLD) is a chronic, debilitating disorder affecting about 30 percent of cotton mill workers and, in later stages, is recognized by the radiographic picture shown in Figure 13. Prior to Dr. Sleeper's pioneering work, early recognition of PDLD was possible only with computed tomography of the chest.

In Dr. Sleeper's study, all 150 workers at the Southern Arizona Pajama Company were scanned using the 5.4-T superconducting body magnet in operation at the Catscratch, Arizona Community Hospital. Magnetic spectra characteristic of polka dot cotton fiber were detected in 26 workers. All those with either positive NMR scans or other clinical evidence of PDLD then underwent the definitive chest computed tomographic scan. Dr. Sleeper's data are shown in Table 23. A false-negative NMR scan was obtained in only one of the 21 workers who had PDLD by tomography, for a sensitivity of 95 percent. The positive predictive accuracy for the NMR scan was 77 percent, indicating a high likelihood of PDLD in workers with a positive scan. Dr. Sleeper concluded that NMR scanning provides a highly sensitive, noninvasive screening test for the early detection of pulmonary polka dots.

Results of a Large Screening Program for PDLD. Corroboration for Dr. Sleeper's work was immediately forthcoming in the research of Dr. J. Birch, company physician for the monolithic Orange County Flag and Bunting Company, which employs several thousand cotton workers. Dr. Birch conducted a study in which 800 patients with confirmed cases of PDLD and 1,700 normal controls were all scanned using NMR. Cases were identified using the criteria of moderate exertional dyspnea, resting hypoxemia ($Pa\text{O}_2 < 65$ mmHg), and chest tomography di-

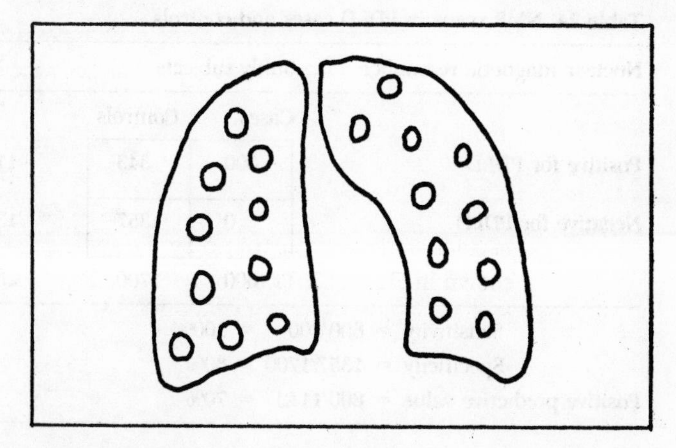

Figure 13. Radiographic appearance of the lungs in polka dot lung disease.

Table 23. Results of NMR scan by results of tomography in cotton pajama workers

Nuclear magnetic resonance	Chest tomography		
	PDLD	Normal	
PDLD	20	6	26
Normal	1	24	25
	21	30	51

Sensitivity = 20/21 = 95%
Specificity = 24/30 = 80%
Positive predictive value = 20/26 = 77%

Table 24. NMR scans in PDLD cases and controls

Nuclear magnetic resonance	Study subjects		
	Cases	Controls	
Positive for PDLD	800	343	1143
Negative for PDLD	0	1357	1357
	800	1700	2500

Sensitivity = 800/800 = 100%
Specificity = 1357/1700 = 80%
Positive predictive value = 800/1143 = 70%

agnostic of PDLD. Controls were free of pulmonary symptoms and signs and had a negative tomogram. Dr. Birch's results are displayed in Table 24.

On the basis of these studies, the International Union of Cotton Workers and Elevator Operators called for the introduction of NMR screening programs in each of the country's 5,347 cotton mills. Claiming a potential for prevention of 50,000 new cases of polka dot lung disease per year, the Government Office for Occupational Safety Evaluation (GOOSE) is funding an emergency program to accelerate production of superconducting body magnets. Plans currently call for diagnostic NMR centers in all cotton factories and on any farm planting more than 20 acres of cotton per year.

Comment

Enthusiasm for new diagnostic tests can often be swift and short-sighted. In the period following the introduction of a new method for diagnosing a disease, the medical literature may be overrun with enthusiastic advocates of the new procedure, test, or instrument. Wary readers must keep in mind the very human, but sometimes mistaken, inclination to embrace uncritically the newest approach or the latest test. Most of us are easy targets for the heartfelt testimony of the Diagnostic Zealot.

Drs. Sleeper and Birch have committed two of the most common errors in the evaluation of diagnostic tests: conducting workups of different intensity in patients with different clinical presentations and evaluating the test in too narrow a clinical spectrum of disease. In Dr. Sleeper's study, only those workers with either a positive NMR scan or "other clinical evidence of PDLD" received the definitive diagnostic procedure (chest tomography). A positive scan caused the investigator to look more intensely for the disease, while a negative scan prompted no further workup in the majority of cases. The diagnostic test (NMR) influenced the depth and completeness of the subsequent workup. Such an approach will usually make a diagnostic test look more sensitive than it really is.

When Dr. Sleeper returned to the factory and completed tomography on the remaining workers not previously studied, the data shown in Table 25 were obtained. The number of false negative NMR scans had markedly increased, from 1 to 30, and the sensitivity of the test had therefore fallen, from 95 percent to 40 percent. A large number of workers with PDLD were missed by NMR scanning, but this was not apparent until the entire population had received equally thorough workups. Our impression of the test as a screening procedure withers a bit.

But what about Dr. Birch's results? He has eliminated the problem of workup bias by having previously completed tomograms on the entire study population. However, Dr. Birch has biased his results by confining his evaluation to a very narrow spectrum of disease. Each of his cases of PDLD is a worker who is desperately ill; this is ensured by the rigorous diagnostic criteria he used. We don't need NMR to diagnose a cotton worker who is blue and breathless.

Although there are others, two of the criteria that should be applied to studies that evaluate diagnostic tests are:

1. Has the diagnostic workup confirming either the presence or absence of the disease been pursued equally in patients with both positive and negative test results? Remember that the sensitivity of this test will be strongly influenced by the intensity of the subsequent search for the disease.
2. Has the test been evaluated in a group of patients who represent a fairly broad spectrum of the disease's clinical and pathological manifestations? Including only patients with advanced or more severe disease can ar-

Table 25. Results of NMR scan by results of tomography in pajama workers (second study)

Nuclear magnetic resonance	Chest tomography		
	PDLD	Normal	
PDLD	20	6	26
Normal	30	94	124
	50	100	150

Sensitivity = 20/50 = 40%
Specificity = 94/100 = 94%
Positive predictive value = 20/26 = 77%

tificially inflate the efficacy of the test in identifying the disease.

Listen cautiously to the earnest jabbering of the Diagnostic Zealot. He sincerely believes all of what he says.

EXAMPLES

Eikman, E. A., Cameron, J. L., Colman, M., et al. A test for patency of the cystic duct in acute cholecystitis. *Am. J. Intern. Med.* 83:318, 1975.

Patients with a positive scan for cholecystitis underwent further investigation, whereas those with a negative scan did not.

Ennis, J. T., Walsh, M. J., and Mahon, J. M. Value of infarct-specific isotope (^{99m}Tc-labeled stannous pyrophosphate) in myocardial scanning. *Br. Med. J.* 3:517, 1975.

Ross, S., Rodriguez, W., Controni, G. Limulus lysate test for gram-negative bacterial meningitis: Bedside application. *J.A.M.A.* 233:1366, 1975.

These are two examples of studies in which the sensitivity of the diagnostic test may be affected by the severity of the disease. Thus, the efficacy of radionucleotide scanning for myocardial infarction may be strongly determined by the size of the infarct; similarly, the accuracy of the limulus lysate test might be a function, in part, of the severity of the gram-negative meningitis. However, the authors do not discuss the grading of disease severity in either case, so the extent of the problem is unknown.

SUGGESTED READING

Ransohoff, D. F., and Feinstein, A. R. Problems of spectrum and bias in evaluating the efficacy of diagnostic tests. *N. Engl. J. Med.* 299:926, 1978.

This is a brief review with examples from the medical literature.

Sackett, D. L. How to read clinical journals: II. To learn about a diagnostic test. *Can. Med. Assoc. J.* 124:703, 1981.

This is another article in Sackett's excellent series on critical analyses of literature; written for clinicians.

A FINAL WORD

Despite their occasional charms, the beasts described here have few friends. The canny researcher will avoid as many of these beasts as he can manage. Those that can't be avoided should be placed under constant surveillance. You might conclude that the value of a research project goes up as the number of beasts goes down; however, it isn't so simple. Medical research is as much an art as medical practice. Splendid investigations have been accomplished despite the messy presence of a bias or two. Conversely, pristine study designs administered under antiseptic conditions can produce drivel. Learning to recognize the beasts is only the first step in weighing the value of a study. Don't let the presence or absence of a few beasts blind you to those qualities of judgment, insight, and an original turn of mind that are the true hallmarks of good science.

association An observed relation between two factors; that is, a tendency for two factors to occur together or to change together. Association is an important criterion for assuming causation. However, not all factors that are associated are causally related.

bias Non-random error; for example, a consistent underestimate in measurement. Not related to the use of the word *bias*, in the sense of prejudice.

cohort A defined group of study subjects, often of similar age, and usually followed over time.

confounding The process by which non-causal association between two factors is produced by association with a third factor known as the confounder. *See* Chap. 1, Grand Confounder.

correlation An association; also, a mathematically defined expression of the strength of an association.

double-blind A condition in which allocation of treatment in experimental studies is unknown to both the experimenter and subject until completion of the study. Observational studies may also be blinded in various ways; for example, interviewers in a case-control study may not be told whether subjects are cases or controls.

endemic The presence of a disease in a defined population at a steady level.

epidemic The outbreak of a disease in a defined population above the level ordinarily expected.

GLOSSARY

epidemiology The study of causes of disease through observations of the distribution of disease among groups of people.

incidence The occurrence of new cases of a given disease in a defined population over a given time period.

mean A way to summarize a set of numbers, calculated by summing individual values and dividing by the total number in the set.

median A way to summarize a set of numbers, represented by the point below and above which 50 percent of values are found (that is, the fiftieth percentile).

mode A way to summarize a set of numbers, represented by the most frequently occurring number in the set.

negative predictive value The probability that a person who is identified by a diagnostic test as healthy, really is healthy; that is, the probability of a "true negative." *See also* Positive predictive value, Sensitivity, Specificity.

odds ratio A measure of risk, usually obtained from case-control studies and (when studying rare diseases) mathematically close to relative risk.

***p*-value** A statistical estimate of the probability that a finding is due to chance. By convention, a finding with a *p*-value less than five percent, or sometimes one percent, is called "statistically significant."

population Any defined group of persons (not necessarily *all* people).

positive predictive value The probability that a person who is identified by a diagnostic test as diseased, really is diseased; that is, the probability of a "true positive." *See also* Negative predictive value, Sensitivity, Specificity.

power The probability that a given study will find a real association to be statistically significant*See* Chap. 10, Nerd of Nonsignificance.

prevalence The proportion of persons with a given disease in a given population at one point in time. Compare with Incidence.

random selection A manner of selecting people for study, in which each person in a defined population has an equal chance of being chosen. Not to be confused with "haphazard."

relative risk A ratio of two risks, expressing their relative size in a single number. Also known as "risk ratio."

reliability The probability that a test or a measure will provide the same result on repeated measurements.

secular Describing a trend over time, as in "a secular decline in heart disease mortality."

sensitivity The probability that a person with a given disease will be correctly classified by some diagnostic test.

specificity The probability that a person without a given disease will be correctly classified by a diagnostic test.

statistical significance A description of results for which it has been estimated mathematically that the chance of the result occurring accidentally is less than five percent, or sometimes one percent. *See also p*-value.

stratification A general strategy for dealing with a variable that may be a confounder, in which subjects are separated into groups according to their level of the confounding variable, and analyzed within those groups. An example of stratification is found in Matchmaker (Chap. 14).

validity The extent to which the results of a study or a measurement correspond to what is actually happening.

Campbell, S. K. *Flaws and Fallacies in Statistical Thinking.* Englewood Cliffs, New Jersey: Prentice-Hall, 1974.

Feinstein, A. R. *Clinical Biostatistics.* St. Louis: Mosby, 1977.

Fletcher, R. H., Fletcher, S. W., and Wagner, E. H. *Clinical Epidemiology: The Essentials.* Baltimore: Williams and Wilkins, 1982.

Friedman, G. D. *Primer of Epidemiology.* New York: McGraw-Hill, 1974.

Gehlbach, S. H. *Interpreting the Medical Literature.* Lexington, MA: Collomore, 1982.

Hill, A. B. *Principles of Medical Statistics.* New York: Oxford University Press, 1971.

Huck, S. W., and Sandler, H. M. *Rival Hypotheses: Alternative Interpretations of Data Based Conclusions.* New York: Harper & Row, 1979.

Kleinbaum, D. G., Kupper, L. L., and Morgenstem, H. *Epidemiologic Research: Principles and Quantitative Methods.* Belmont, CA: Lifetime Learning, 1982.

BIBLIOGRAPHY

Last, J. M. *A Dictionary of Epidemiology*. New York: Oxford University Press, 1983.

Lilienfeld, A. M., and Lilienfeld, D. E. *Foundations of Epidemiology* (2nd ed.). New York: Oxford University Press, 1980.

MacMahon, B., and Pugh, T. F. *Epidemiology: Principles and Methods*. Boston: Little, Brown, 1970.

Mausner, J. S., and Bahn, A. K. *Epidemiology: An Introductory Text*. Philadelphia: Saunders, 1974.

Morris, J. N. *Uses of Epidemiology*. Edinburgh: Churchill Livingston, 1974.

Riegelman, R. K. *Studying a Study and Testing a Test: How to Read the Medical Literature*. Boston: Little, Brown, 1981.

Susser, M. *Causal Thinking in the Health Sciences*. New York: Oxford University Press, 1973.

INDEX